THE LITTLE POCKET BOOK OF

STRETCHING
WITH EASE FOR A
PAIN-FREE BACK

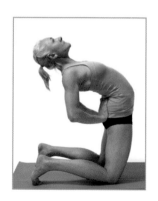

T0162238

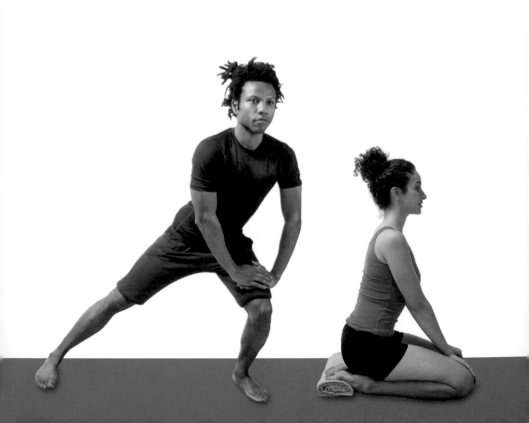

THE LITTLE POCKET BOOK OF

STRETCHING
WITH EASE FOR A
PAIN-FREE BACK

heal and prevent backache and injury

LINDA MINARIK

CICO BOOKS

LONDON NEW YORK

For Dalmo and Dan, who always believed in me.
And for my Dad, in gratitude for his love and bravery.

Published in 2017 by CICO Books
an imprint of Ryland Peters & Small Ltd
20–21 Jockey's Fields, London WC1R 4BW
341 E 116th St, New York, NY 10029

www.rylandpeters.com

The material in this book was previously published by
CICO Books in 2015 as part of *Stretching with Ease*.

10 9 8 7 6 5 4 3 2 1

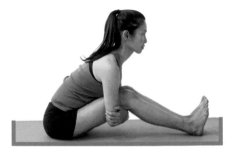

A CIP catalog record for this book is available from the
Library of Congress and the British Library.

ISBN: 978-1-78249-527-7

Printed in China

Editor: Jane Birch
Designer: Emily Breen
Design concept: Isobel Gillan
Photographer and illustrator: Rob Zeller

Commissioning editor: Kristine Pidkameny
Senior editor: Carmel Edmonds
Art director: Sally Powell
Production controller: Mai-Ling Collyer
Publishing manager: Penny Craig
Publisher: Cindy Richards

Please note that the information in this book should
not be substituted for advice from your physician. If
you have any health concerns, consult your physician
for guidance before doing any of the exercises in this
book. The publisher and the author cannot be held
responsible for any health issue that may arise
indirectly or directly from the use of this book.

contents

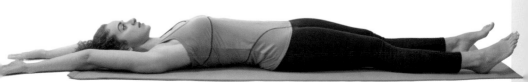

introduction

After we've got to the bottom of an issue, and we've gained some perspective about the crisis it has caused, the solution seems simple. That's retrospect. But, when we're in the middle of that issue and a successful conclusion does not seem inevitable, it's a mystery. Back pain can be like this. Where do we look for help?

Think about how you feel when faced with pain. A strong enough pain leaves you no room to think of anything except getting rid of it. A very strong pain brings the word "desperation" to mind. It can seem mundane to try a simple technique like stretching when desire for instant relief consumes you. However, think about this: often pain tells you that the body has reached its strength limit as it tried to function in some imbalanced position. The painful area of the body is probably under long-standing stress from compensation, and muscles may actually be in spasm, unable to let go and relax. Stretching is therefore a great little resource to have in your personal array of remedies.

Elsewhere in this book you will find several perspectives on and ideas for releasing pain (Why Stretch?, Benefit 3, pp. 17–18; and Stretch To Relieve Common Areas of Pain, pp. 144–151). But the absolute most important thing, once your pain has lessened enough to free your mind for other

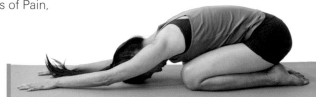

questions, is to locate that imbalance and correct it. Figure it out and enlist your personal team of knowledgeable and trusted professionals. This is a slightly longer-term project, but the most effective one if you want permanent freedom from pain. Use your creativity and your body's signals (they're there if you tune in!), because the person who knows your body best—and is thus best suited to fathom its mystery—is *you*.

WHAT IS FLEXIBILITY?

Flexibility is the freedom we have to move with as great a range of motion, in all our body parts, as we need for any activity we want to undertake. In other words:

- For daily life you need enough flexibility to bend down and pick up something you dropped on the floor.

- For aerobic dance you need enough flexibility to lift your knee to 90 degrees without tucking your pelvis under.

- For gymnastics you need enough flexibility to execute a split.

Whatever you want to accomplish—however simple or complex the movement—possessing adequate flexibility means you can do it easily, without a struggle. Stretching is what you do to acquire that flexibility.

What you will find here is a jumping-off place for your personal research. You will get enough information to provide you with a mental foothold as you begin to explore using flexibility to bring some benefit into your life—but not enough information to overwhelm you. You do not need any previous experience with stretching to employ the knowledge presented here. If you are already an experienced stretching practitioner, the clear instructions offered can help you organize the knowledge you have, and maybe give you some ideas for the next steps in your quest for ever-greater freedom of movement.

SOME THINGS TO CONSIDER AS YOU BEGIN

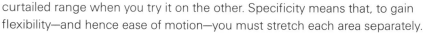

- **Flexibility is specific.** If you can bend over and put your palms on the ground, that's great, but it doesn't guarantee that you can open your knees wide to the side in a kneeling position. You may have a fairly good range of motion when you do a stretch on one side of your body, and a curtailed range when you try it on the other. Specificity means that, to gain flexibility—and hence ease of motion—you must stretch each area separately.

- **Equally, remember that your body is an interconnected and complex system.** Most of us would go straight for the stretches that directly target the back. Seems logical, right? But, often, an imbalance at a site distant from the actual pain location can be the culprit. That is why this book also includes stretches for the abdominals, hips, and thighs. Releasing muscular tightness in one or more of these areas may well be key to a successfully solved mystery. Don't underestimate the power of a side hip stretch when addressing a sacrum issue.

IN CONCLUSION

Your experience is your own—and only your own. Never discount its validity. No one can know what will benefit you better than you do. Ask advice of others; consult books like this one. When all the evidence is in, the best decisions about how to proceed are rightfully yours.

Consider using the stretches provided here in the spirit of research. How can I make my body feel better? What ideal stretching recipe will I discover? Happy exploring!

CONVENTIONS USED IN PART TWO: YOUR
STRETCH REPERTORY

- **Sports injury list.** At the beginning of each chapter in this section is a selection of sports injuries that the stretches discussed might help to heal. The list is not comprehensive; neither are the injuries defined. They are terms in common use, and will be familiar to many readers. The injuries mentioned will be most relevant if you have been "diagnosed" with one of these conditions as a result of pain in an area: you will recognize the name and be able to use the appropriate stretches.

- **Stretch descriptions.** We describe each of the 39 stretches referenced in this section for one side of your body only. All tips and thoughts are oriented to this first side. When you stretch the other side, just switch the words "right" and "left."

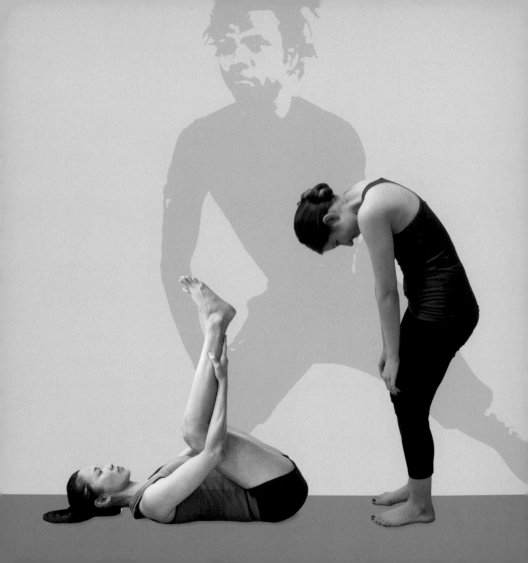

PART ONE:
BEFORE YOU STRETCH

You are the master of the partnership between your body and your mind. Like many people who take my flexibility classes, you are pursuing excellent personal fitness. Perhaps you are not a professional in fitness, but you are certainly a professional elsewhere in your life. You have job experience that is irreplaceable, or a combination of personal and workplace qualities shared by no one else. Acknowledge your unique qualities, and bring them to flexibility training. This group of articles will introduce you to some solid logic behind the study of stretching. Get your discerning mind behind learning how to stretch correctly and well, and you will increase your chances of successfully—and permanently—incorporating a beneficial flexibility practice into your life. I hope that the material in this section will afford you the right impetus to launch that practice.

why stretch?

Why would you take time from an incredibly busy life for a slow activity like stretching? Life is full of demands on every side. Many professional people start work early and get home late. Busy mothers find their days broken up by driving kids to multiple activities. Time is at a premium—for everyone. Entertain the possibility that inserting a stretch and a breath into an odd free moment can make all the hustle seem less hectic.

Our days of hunting and gathering, and spending our days tracking, killing, and cooking food—or else outrunning the proverbial saber-toothed tiger—may be behind us, but the myth that modern conveniences make our fast-paced, worldwide-web lives simpler is just that: a myth.

We no longer have to fear becoming a tiger's dinner, but there are still plenty of tiger stand-ins around to trigger our fight-or-flight responses. And our systems are hardwired: they react the same way to a high-pressure work deadline as they would to a prehistoric tiger.

The techniques you will learn in this book have the capacity to take you farther along the road to true relaxation than you would get by merely stretching a muscle or only quieting the mind. By joining thought, body awareness, and movement, it is possible to create a space inside yourself where the pressures bearing on you do not exist. Even if you can spare only ten minutes, choosing techniques from those offered that benefit your unique makeup most can be enough to dissipate the negative effects of stress, help to prevent injury, relieve pain and muscular soreness, improve your posture and level of well-being, and up your athletic ability. Life will still be there when you emerge from your stretching space, but you will be much better equipped to face it.

I invite you to create an interior magic bubble where life's overriding concerns are unable to reach you. Although you cannot recover or replace the precious resource of time, I invite you to devote a little of the time you have to something that has the potential to make the rest of it calmer, better-feeling, and more efficient: stretching.

Benefit 1: stretching reduces and heals stress

Stress is a very real "aging" agent. Negative stress in its many incarnations is alive and well and with us in the 21st century, as the briefest glance at your life will show. And one thing you can do to counteract its evil effects is—stretch.

For the body to increase its range of muscle movement, it must calm down. Your body is very often in "alert" mode, constantly looking over its shoulder, so to speak, to make sure it is safe. Such a never-ending state of stress does not advance optimum health. But how can you dissipate this state? Just see what happens when you put your body into a flexibility class, lie down on the floor, and use the exhale phase of your breath to allow a particular muscle to relax and lengthen. When you exhale, your body gets the message, "It is safe to relax. I am in a safe place." Your body can start to open up and increase its muscular range—but not if it isn't convinced it has nothing to fear. By definition, when the body is able to increase muscle range of movement, your nervous system uses the parasympathetic—relaxing—branch of the autonomic nervous system (ANS). You are less likely to trigger the go-on-alert branch of the ANS—the sympathetic. You experience fewer detrimental effects from stress. Your stress level goes down.

Benefit 2: stretching prevents injury

Injury prevention—a pair of words you might struggle to get your mind around. These words have been used so often they may border on useless jargon. Here's a simple situation you can envision.

At some time in your life you may have done something called "twisting your ankle." Accidentally, of course. It takes you unawares. Suddenly you're on the floor in pain, and you end up with a swollen ankle. In my high school basketball days, I was so familiar with this situation that I actually started wearing ACE™ bandages over my ankles to every practice.

The ankle always turns on the outside of your foot—never the inside. Try this. Stand with your feet side by side and let your right ankle drop outside—to the right. It goes over rather easily. Now drop it inside—to the left. It doesn't go there, right? The ankle has much more tendency to collapse out than in. That's your vulnerable spot.

Now, let's say you did the following stretch twice a week for two months.

Sit down in a chair and place your right ankle on your left thigh. Let your right knee open. Now, gently stretch the right ankle into the "turned-ankle" position and hold for 30 seconds. Experience the stretchy feeling, but stop short of actual pain. No forcing. Repeat three times. Then repeat on the other ankle. Your investment of time for this is about five minutes. You can do it while you are (famously) watching TV.

The next time you turn your ankle (always a shock), your ankle will be capable of displacing itself farther from its home position without harm. The stretch has prevented an injury.

The same principle applies to other stretches. Think of the golfer's swing and how his spine must twist—both in the wind-up and the release. If the spine rotates on a regular basis, the body will not feel it is doing anything out of the ordinary, and therefore won't injure itself during the move. The philosophy is: don't wait until an injury occurs. Add this new dimension to your fitness program now.

Benefit 3: stretching relieves pain

One important place to experience this effect is in the area of lower-back pain, often exacerbated by tight hamstrings (muscles in the back of your thighs). The lower back and sacrum (spine below your waist) cause many people pain. Although many doctors are of the opinion that the sacral vertebrae are "fused" and operate totally as a unit, there is actually a little movement available in that area.

If people learn techniques to increase that movement ability gently, freeing the vertebrae from constriction while they also loosen up the hamstring muscles, the pain can be reduced or eliminated.

The connection of tight hamstrings with back pain is a good case in point, because tight hamstrings stop the hips from flexing during forward bending, forcing the lower back to bend beyond its strong middle range. This is the sort of thing that may happen in a yoga class, if the teacher is not knowledgeable enough to spot and correct it. The back overstretches to accommodate tight hamstrings, and the problem (and the pain) may just get worse. If you work in an office, the constant chair-sitting you do is already contributing to this problem, even before you add any exercises that work hamstrings—which makes them tighter.

The same principle applies to improving mobility in other areas. Hence, a stretching program can go far toward relieving pain. It can also happen that one part of the body becomes tight, and another part compensates: you feel the tightness in the compensating area. When you stretch one area—such as the upper back—pain may be relieved in another area—such as the lower back.

Benefit 4: stretching relieves muscular soreness
You are probably familiar with what is termed "post-exercise muscle soreness." When you work muscles you are not used to using, or work your muscles at a different angle, they get sore a day or two later. There are dietary measures and supplements you can take to reduce this soreness, but when you do experience it, stretching can come to the rescue.

After reading this book, you will be familiar with what muscles are located where in your body, what it feels like to stretch each particular muscle group, and what stretches to do when you are confronted with muscle soreness in an area. In this respect, you can become your own physical therapist or personal trainer. You will have knowledge that allows you to remedy the little soreness glitches your body may develop as you go along living your life and doing your fitness program of choice.

Benefit 5: stretching improves posture and body symmetry
Your ability to move your body easily in any direction you wish can be impaired by habitual actions, like:

- Emphasis on working only one side of the body—such as arm wrestling. One arm becomes much stronger than the other.

- Emphasis on working one muscle group to the exclusion of another. When bodybuilders emphasize the bench press (chest) more than back exercises, the chest muscles become strong and tight and can round the shoulders forward.

- Sitting with shoulders rounded forward—again shortening the chest muscles and weakening the back muscles that should work to keep the shoulders centered

Working and stretching both sides of the body provide a good solution for situations like these.

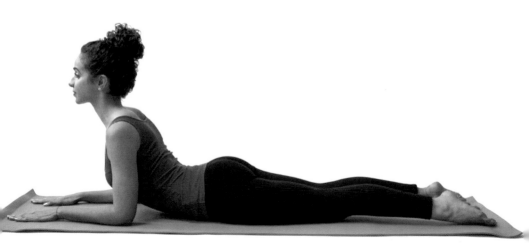

how muscles respond to stretching

Here are a few strategies that respect the characteristic ways your body behaves when it stretches:

- **Stretching each side separately will yield greater range than stretching both sides at once.** You can see this when you do a simple test. Perform the quadriceps stretch 31 (see p. 112) with both legs; then stretch each leg separately. You will probably be able to pull your heel closer to your buttocks when you stretch one leg at a time. Also, contrast stretch 34 (see p. 119), in which both legs stretch together, with stretch 35 (see p. 122), in which one leg stretches at a time. You will probably gain greater pull and range in the back of each thigh when you stretch one thigh at a time than when you must distribute the stretch between both thighs. That's how the body is wired.

- **Stretch the less flexible side first.** Your body tends to give its best effort to the first thing you do. If you know that your left hamstring is less flexible than your right, stretch the left one first. After you do the right side, you can return to the left for some extra time. This will help even out your flexibility range.

- **The body responds with more range of motion when stretches are repeated more than once.** The body is learning what you want it to do, how to become a good partner for your mind as you create your flexible body. It needs a little time to get used to a position, and you will often find that, after a little rest, your body will open up more the second time you do the stretch.

- **Neutralize the stretch reflex.** Whenever a muscle is stretched, its response is to contract. This is why Ballistic Stretching (see box on p. 24) is not recommended—because that's exactly what happens when you stretch by vigorously bouncing. When you stretch to increase range of motion, (a) begin with a completely relaxed muscle, and (b) stretch slowly, taking your time (see Longer Static Stretching, p. 25). This will keep the stretch reflex from occurring, and help you achieve a much greater range of motion in the stretched muscles.

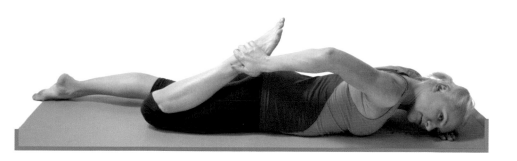

ways to stretch: how to do it

TYPES OF STRETCHING

Books on stretching classify stretching methods according to different rules.

Some authors classify Static Stretching as a separate type from Passive Stretching. There are other subgroups like Passive/Active and Active-Assisted. I prefer a simpler division: Active Stretching and Passive Stretching, with variations on those two main types.

Active stretching

In this method, the muscles opposing the ones stretching are contracting. Example: a front kick, executed with your own muscular power—and then held at the highest point of the kick. The hamstrings (back of the leg) are stretching; the quadriceps (front of the leg) are contracting.

Active Stretching is important for arts and disciplines like ballet and gymnastics. They require the athlete to hold limbs and torso in stationary positions, which are also stretched positions. This book does not discuss this type of Active Stretching. It's mentioned here to show you that flexibility study is a wide world.

Stretch in Motion (see p. 24) and PNF Stretching (see p. 26) use components of Active Stretching, but these do not really fit the strict definition above, since the muscles stretching are the same ones that contract (contract and relax in sequence).

Passive stretching

This basically means that your muscles are not contracting; instead, you do everything you can to get them to relax. Their stretch comes from an outside force. That force can be a trainer or partner assisting with the stretch; a prop such as a towel or wall; or you can supply the force yourself in various ways, such as leaning forward or pulling one body part with another (for example, pulling the fingers of one hand with the other).

This book concentrates on methods of Passive Stretching.

YOUR STRETCHING METHOD CATALOG

Passive Stretching protocols can be classified as some variation of:

1 Moving into and out of a stretch.

2 Holding a stretch position.

3 Using resistance at some point during a stretch.

This section gives you a lexicon of methods that have worked for me, both personally and in my teaching practice.

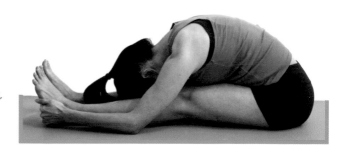

BALLISTIC STRETCHING

The technique of Ballistic Stretching is an older method, now pretty much out of favor. It involves vigorous bouncing in and out of the stretch, which is generally considered to activate the body's "stretch reflex": because of the violence of the movement, the body immediately contracts the muscle you just stretched, and your net flexibility gain is zero.

Moving into and out of a stretch

- **Stretch in Motion.** Here you move into a stretch, then out of it, in rhythm. This does not imply any bouncing, but uses a lift-then-lengthen technique instead.

  Example: To stretch your lower back and sacrum using Stretch in Motion, lie on the floor on your back. Place one hand on each knee, or behind each thigh (see stretch 1a, p. 36). At a moderate breathing tempo, inhale. Exhale and pull your knees toward your chest. Inhale—slightly release the pull; exhale—gently pull your knees in. Continue this rhythmic pull-and-release motion for two sets of eight repetitions.

A common term in use today for this way of stretching is *dynamic* stretching.

- **Rhythmic Breathing.** This is a much slower method of moving into and out of a stretch. On a long, slow exhale, move deeper into the stretch position. On the inhale, decrease the pressure. This doesn't mean you pull out of the stretch— just let up slightly on the intensity. (See also Using the Tool of Breathing, p. 28.)

Example: To stretch your lower back using Rhythmic Breathing, lie on the floor on your back, knees to your chest, with one hand on each knee (see stretch 1a, p. 36). On a long, slow exhale, pull your knees farther in toward your chest; feel your lower back stretch. On the inhale, decrease the strength of your pull, and feel the stretch lessen slightly.

Holding a stretch

I use two variations of this technique: Shorter Static Stretching and Longer Static Stretching. They differ only in the length of time you hold the stretch. Enter the stretch you have chosen; align your body as optimally as you can. Hold the position. Locate the stretchy feeling with your mind. When you feel your body's resistance diminish, move a little farther into the stretch.

- **Shorter Static Stretching.** Hold the stretch for 30 to 45 seconds.

- **Longer Static Stretching.** Hold the stretch for one minute or longer. Depending on your goal and flexibility level, three or four minutes is not unfeasible.

Example: To stretch your buttocks using Shorter Static Stretching, sit on a chair with your right foot on the floor and your left ankle crossed over your right knee (see stretch 20, p. 88). Lift your sacrum and lower back up and out of your hips, begin to lean slowly forward, and keep your back flat. Concentrate on the felt stretch; keep a steady pressure. Hold for 30 to 45 seconds. Repeat on the other side.

Using resistance during a stretch

- **PNF Stretching.** "PNF" stands for Proprioceptive Neuromuscular Facilitation. There are a couple of variations on this technique. I use the following one:

  Place your body in the stretch position you have chosen. Contract the muscle you are stretching as hard as you can—really access it—for a specified length of time. Hold the contraction for eight slow counts, four counts, two—develop your own practice protocol.

  Here is the trick: when your chosen count is complete, relax the muscular contraction, and immediately move a little farther into the stretch position. This does not mean release the position—relax the contraction. There is a split second between the moment you release the contraction and the muscle's relapse into its former degree of stiffness. If you seize that instant—before the

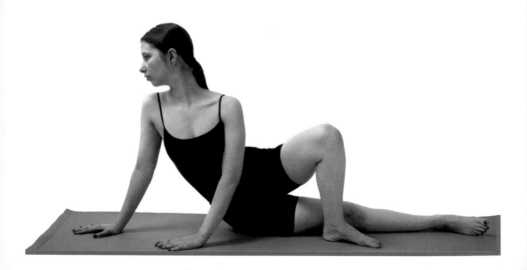

body starts thinking, "Oh, I remember: I'm tight here"—you will gain a quite remarkable increase in range in that muscle. But you must not delay, or you will lose that tiny window of possibility.

This is an intense technique. Repeat several times, designing your own hold variations, depending on how your body feels about doing it.

Example: To stretch your hamstrings using PNF Stretching, stand on your left leg and place your straight right leg onto a chair or a table (see stretch 35, p. 122). Lift your back straight up and away from your legs; lean slowly forward; and keep your back flat. Push your leg down against the surface as hard as you can—the hamstring muscles in the back of your leg will activate. Hold for your chosen count. At the moment you relax the hamstring contraction, see how much farther forward you can lean your flat-back torso into the stretch position. After your chosen number of repetitions, repeat on the other side.

REMEMBER

The goal you have in mind determines the character and duration of the stretch you do.

Note: Not every stretching method is suitable for every stretch. A good instructor can help you match the protocol with the stretch, and also you will develop greater body awareness as you practice flexibility.

using the tool of breathing

Breathing: open the door to flexibility

The passage of oxygen in and out of our lungs is what we call "breathing." Thousands of times a day, every day of our lives, this process goes on. When we want to say that something is part of the fabric of our lives, we say it is "as natural as breathing." Since breathing goes on nonstop, we are not always aware of it, tending to take it for granted. Yet, consider how vital breathing is to our existence. We can live three weeks without food, three days without water, but only three minutes without air (15 minutes at the very outside before brain death).

Breathing is a semiconscious process, which means we have some control over its tempo. Faster breathing signals the body to be on the alert; slower breathing calms it down. This becomes important as we seek to relax and open the body through stretching. If we gasp, or hold our breath, the body goes into survival-alert mode. We have all experienced the involuntary intake of breath triggered by an unexpected event. We are hardwired this way, because survival is our body's first priority. Holding our breath is similar. The body knows its breath-holding limit (30 seconds for the average untrained person), and the clock starts ticking as soon as we forget to exhale. This is not conducive to relaxation. The body has other things on its mind.

The bottom line is: if we want to profit maximally from stretching, we must coax our body to relax. We must convince our body that it is in a safe place, that it is okay for it to let tension go. Correct, conscious stretching is capable of releasing deeply held, tight areas in the body—of which we may not even be aware until we feel and release them. But if we don't breathe deeply and slowly, the body just will not open. Breathing is your ticket to stretching success.

HOW TO USE IT

For most methods of stretching, paying attention to breathing slowly and deeply, without gasping or holding the breath, is sufficient. Spend a few moments noticing how you breathe naturally. Do you lift your shoulders when you breathe? Do you expand your abdomen as well as your chest when you breathe? Or do you not expand anywhere at all?

See if you can take a good, full breath that widens your ribcage without lifting your shoulders. Your chest will also deepen a little. Once you experience ribcage and chest expansion, see if you can add abdominal relaxation and increase its space as well. On the exhale, the ribcage and chest deflate again, and you can contract your abdomen slightly as the breath leaves that area.

It might be a good idea to take a few minutes before your stretch practice to familiarize your body with this enhanced way of breathing. In the thick of your session, especially when you are learning new techniques, you may forget to breathe like this. But, as repetition makes the concepts and movements more familiar to you, it will be easier to hold more than one thing in your mind.

This basic, heightened-breathing method is appropriate for the following stretching techniques:

- Shorter Static Stretching.

- Longer Static Stretching.

- PNF Stretching (see p. 26).

Stretch in Motion
This method presents a slightly different case. You will likely be using Stretch in Motion as part of a warm-up to prepare your body for a vigorous activity, so your breathing tempo will naturally increase. Just keep your shoulders relaxed as you let the breath flow in and out.

Rhythmic Breathing
The case of Rhythmic Breathing (see p. 24) is somewhat different again. Here you move more deeply into the stretch on your long, slow exhale, and relax the intensity of your position on the inhale. By joining a very slight motion with the timing

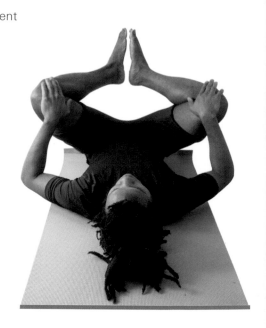

of your breathing, and adding concentration, you can tune in to the smallest variations in muscular feeling. By mentally "cocking an ear" to your body's reactions as you hold the stretch, you can respond instantly—a little more pressure, a little less. You can feel tiny changes in your body's tension and relaxation levels. It is possible to merge so completely with your body that you approach a meditative state.

In terms of inducing your body to relax, Rhythmic Breathing is a star in your arsenal of tools. What it really does is trick your body into sinking more deeply into a stretch. From your body's point of view, it knows you are going to ask for an intense stretch during one exhale only. Then it will get a break when you inhale and slightly release the pressure. So it will likely go there for you. However, note the degree of stretch your muscles have before you do this technique and check again afterward. Probably you have sneakily wheedled your body into increasing its range—behind its back, as it were.

You might want to plan a certain number of breaths to complete during a particular stretch. For example, try ten breaths and see what results you get.

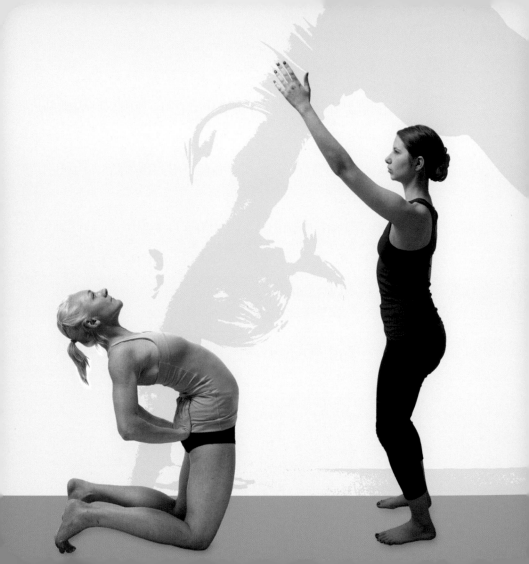

PART TWO

YOUR STRETCH REPERTORY

Delve into the ingredient mix for your stretching program—an organized list of stretches at a glance. Here we get down to brass tacks with the basics. How can you allow your body to release gently into a stretch? How can you align yourself correctly so other body areas do not become stressed? And—crucial to your stretching education—exactly where should you be feeling muscular pull? The instructions emphasize giving your body enough time to settle into a position, without rushing into or out of it. A unique plus: increase your sense of calm and minimize fear by creating a partnership between your mind and your body. You will learn to recruit your mind to address your body's tight spots.

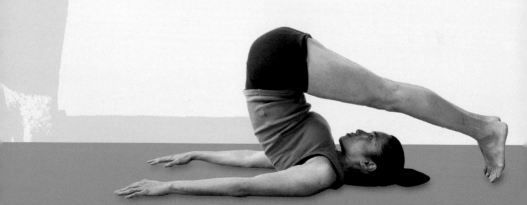

BACK

In this section we will cover stretches for the lower and upper back, both in flexion and extension, as well as lengthening moves that encompass the full spine. During each technique, look for the feeling of stretch in the areas described.

PELVIC TUCK AND TILT: WHAT'S THE DIFFERENCE?

What *is* the difference? Lie on your back on the floor, knees bent and feet on the floor. Tuck your pelvis: flatten your lower-back curve against the floor. There will be no space between you and the floor all along your back, and your pubic bone will lift up toward your chest. Tilt your pelvis: push your pubic bone down and away from you, and feel that your butt is sticking out. The curve in your lower back returns, and gets bigger. (Keep your ribs on the floor, so that only the pelvis moves.) Now relax everything, and you are in pelvic neutral— neither tucked nor tilted.

Causes of stiff, sore, or aching back muscles/ muscles in spasm

....

Injuries eased by stretching

....

Additional uses

- A whole day of maintaining the upright or sitting position, which compresses spinal discs and pushes the cushioning fluid out from between them.
- Sitting at the computer—or any long sitting session, such as attending a business conference.
- Playing sports—almost any sport requires constant back use. Examples are basketball, cycling, racquetball/handball, running, swimming, walking, and yoga.
- Any intense or prolonged exercise.

. . . .

- Upper- or lower-back muscle strain (choose appropriate stretch).
- Upper- or lower-back ligament sprain (mild) (choose appropriate stretch).
- Abdominal muscle strain (obliques, stretch 13).

. . . .

- Before and after playing sports requiring constant or intense back movement, including twisting movements—basketball, cycling, racquetball/handball, running, swimming, walking.
- When you wake up still tired with a nagging backache. Your muscles may be too stiff to allow spine decompression as you sleep.

Pinpoint the area of discomfort (this connects your mind with your body), and choose the stretch that most closely reaches that spot. **For guidance on stretch duration, see p. 25. To discover how to use breathing to deepen the stretch, see pp. 28–31.**

1a lower back (flexion): knees to chest

These three stretches are a progression from the least intense to the most intense. If you are in pain or just beginning your flexibility training, you would probably start with stretch 1a. As your back feels better or you gain more flexibility, you can move to 1b. Stretch 1c, The Plough, requires the most flexibility. In my own case, there was a long summer when I practiced it almost every morning. At the end of the summer I achieved the plough. Moral? With stretching, patience in practice pays off.

- **The Setup:** Lie on a comfortable but supportive surface, such as a carpet or an exercise mat. A bed doesn't provide enough support for your body, although you can wake yourself up with modified versions of some stretches before getting out of bed in the morning (see Upon Waking in the Morning, p. 158).
  Make sure the back of your neck is nice and long. This means your chin will be more tucked into your chest than pointed to the ceiling. Cultivate the feeling that some friendly hand is pulling the base of your skull gently along the floor, allowing a long, free feeling to appear in the back of your neck.

- **The Stretch:** Place one hand on each knee (or behind each thigh) and pull your knees toward your chest. Look for a feeling of length in the muscles of your spine below your waist—your sacrum.

- **Enhance Your Flexibility:** Feel how the stretch changes as you alternately slowly sink your butt to the floor and allow it to rise again slightly—without moving your knees. This is good movement education for your sacral muscles.

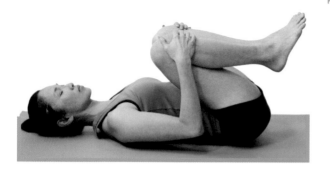

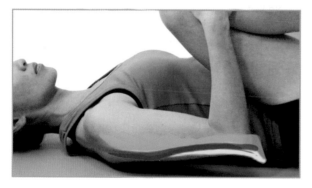

As you pull your knees into your chest, allow your body to become very heavy and really sink into the floor. Neck longer, back so heavy it even goes through the floor. Even though you are stretching your lower back/sacral area, allowing other muscles to release contractions, you may not be aware of can increase your general relaxation.

Note: These muscles lie underneath the arm but, for the purposes of illustration, the muscles are shown overlaying the arm. All muscles shown are stretching on both sides of the body.

KEY TO MUSCLES
Erector spinae:
Iliocostalis
Longissimus cervicis, thoracis
Spinalis thoracis

Multifidi

1b lower back (flexion): lower legs extended

- **The Setup:** Lie on your back on a comfortable—but not-too-soft—surface. Keep your neck long and supple, with your chin not quite tucked—but definitely not pointing toward the ceiling.

- **The Stretch:** Begin by pulling your knees gently into your chest. Either use one hand on each knee, or one hand behind each thigh—whichever position is more comfortable for you. (This is the 1a position.) It is okay to allow your butt to lift slightly off the floor.

  Placing one hand on each calf, begin to unfold your lower legs. With your knees still bent, pull the calves toward you. This will make your thighs come closer to your chest, exerting a more intense pull on your lower-back/sacrum area. As you become more flexible, you will be able to adjust your hands on your calves to the position that will give you the greatest degree of possible stretch.

- **Enhance Your Flexibility:** Stretching on your back with the knees bent emphasizes the lower-back/sacrum stretch, with minimum involvement of the backs of your legs (hamstrings). Pay attention to how this variation increases the stretchy feeling (intensity) compared to 1a.

KEY TO MUSCLES
Erector spinae:

Iliocostalis

Longissimus cervicis, thoracis

Spinalis thoracis

Multifidi

Note: These muscles lie underneath the arm but, for the purposes of illustration, the muscles are shown overlaying the arm. All muscles shown are stretching on both sides of the body.

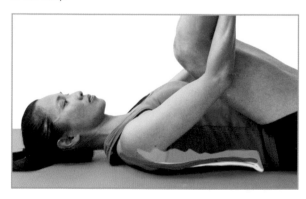

ENLIST YOUR MIND

A clear mental concept always helps your stretching progress. Sure knowledge of what and where the sacrum and lower back actually are will serve you much better than vague ideas about their location. This is particularly important because the back is behind you. Human orientation is naturally focused toward the front, so what's in back is more challenging for us to sense. It is possible to delve into fine detail on this point but, simply put, your lower back is in the area of your waistline. Your belly button is opposite your lumbar (lower-back) vertebrae— in the range of L3 to L5. The sacrum is below that— basically the pelvic area.

1c lower back (flexion): legs over head

- **The Setup:** As in stretches 1a and 1b, lie on your back on a supportive and comfortable surface. Your neck is long, your chin sinking slightly toward your chest.

- **The Stretch:** Here, since this is the most intense of our lower-back/sacrum flexion series, begin as in 1a by pulling your knees gently into your chest, using your preferred hand position—on your knee or behind your thigh. Intensify the stretch by passing through 1b: unfold your lower legs and gently press your thighs toward your chest.

  An optimally executed 1c stretch is close to your maximum lower-back flexion range. You may take many incremental steps on your way to this goal.

  Begin to move into 1c from 1b by giving your butt a push to lift it and take it backward. If you don't need to push with your arms, use your core to bring your bent legs up and over your head. Slowly straighten your legs. The stretchy feeling will increase simultaneously in the backs of your legs and in your lower-back/sacrum area. Hold for your chosen duration; then slowly bend your knees again and return, through stretch 1b, to your original position with knees to chest.

- **Enhance Your Flexibility:** Once you are able to straighten your legs, you can increase your range by gently holding onto your legs, wherever you can reach, and pulling them in the direction of your ears.

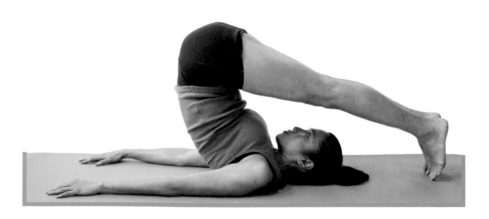

Monitor your chin. Identify the shortening feeling in the back of your neck when the chin starts creeping up to the ceiling. Spare it half a thought—and then adjust it downward to relax the back of the neck. Develop this wider sense of body position. As you do, it will become second nature.

KEY TO MUSCLES

Erector spinae:

■ Longissimus thoracis
▨ Iliocostalis

▢ Semitendinosus
■ Biceps femoris (long head)
■ Biceps femoris (short head)

Note: All muscles shown are stretching on both sides of the body.

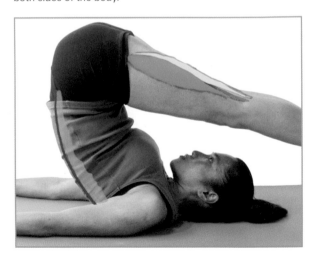

2 lower back (flexion):
chest to thighs, kneeling

- **The Setup:** This stretch is the flip side of stretch 1a, "Knees to Chest." It carries a bit more intensity than the first stretch, because your body weight is now pressing your chest closer to your thighs, which creates more length in your back than you can get by pulling your knees into your chest, as in stretch 1a.
  Start by kneeling on the floor and open your knees a bit. Flatten your feet (toes are not tucked on this one).

- **The Stretch:** Let your butt sink back toward your heels. See how far back you can take your butt. You have gained a good amount of flexibility when you feel your butt touching your heels.
  Choose your arm and head position: (1) reach your arms forward and place your forehead on the floor; (2) cross your elbows in front of you and rest your

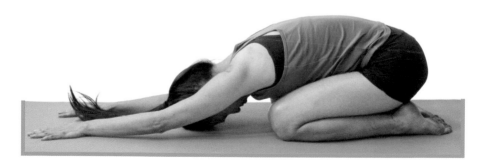

forehead on your forearms; or (3) position your
arms at your sides and rest your forehead on
the floor.

• **Enhance Your Flexibility:** See if you can locate
your sacrum using your inside radar and gently
flatten it, so that your abdomen and chest come
closer to your thighs. This will increase the stretch
and develop awareness of sacral movement. If you
can sense your sacrum and lower back moving
up and away from your hips and legs, your ability
to flex your spine farther and farther forward
will grow. This feeling is a tool you can use to
overcome stiffness and create a fluid lower-back/
hamstring connection.

Note: All muscles shown are
stretching on both sides of
the body.

KEY TO MUSCLES
Erector spinae:
▉ Iliocostalis
▉ Longissimus
▉ Spinalis thoracis

▉ Multifidi

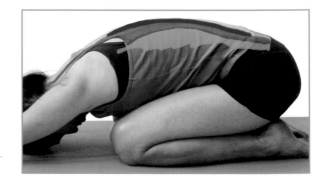

3 lower back (flexion):
backward pull, seated

- **The Setup:** Here you are still targeting the same muscles you lengthened in stretches 1a–c and stretch 2. You may find one stretch more effective than another, because every body is different. In this lower-back/sacrum stretch group you have several choices to try out.

    This particular position uses your body's own leverage to create the stretchy feeling.

    Sit on the floor with both legs straight out in front of you. Flex both feet; bend your knees slightly; open your toes to the side. If you were to stand up, you would be using Charlie Chaplin's signature pose, or standing in the first position in ballet, with a little plié.

- **The Stretch:** Grab your heels with your hands. It's fine if you cannot reach your heels: just hold onto your legs as far down as you can without too much discomfort. Keeping a firm grip on your heels or legs, drop your head down between your arms and relax your neck. Your view is your belly button.

    Lean gently back, away from the pull of your hands. Look for the stretchy feeling, as before, in the area of your waistline and below. Slow pulsing or static holding work well with this stretch (see Part One: Ways to Stretch, p. 22).

- **Enhance Your Flexibility:** This stretch, more than the others in the section, has a specific focus at the waistline. When you first experience its power, you may realize that your back has been asleep in this spot. Wake it up with care. Judge how much pull to exert, as your body settles in and learns how to feel this stretch.

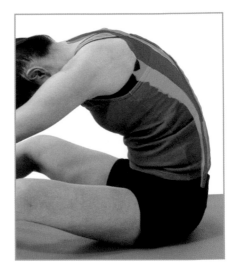

Note: All muscles shown are stretching on both sides of the body.

KEY TO MUSCLES
Erector spinae:
- Iliocostalis
- Longissimus
- Spinalis thoracis

- Multifidi

4 lower back (flexion):
hug and release, seated

The photographs for this setup and stretch are on the following page.

- **The Setup:** Sit on the floor with your knees bent and feet in front of you. Hug your elbows around your thighs; grab each opposite elbow with your hands. Pull your chest right to the thighs. Bend your knees as much as you need to in order to feel your chest actually touching your thighs. You may already be experiencing the lifting-up feeling in your lower-back/sacral area. Relax your head forward so you do not tax the neck muscles.

- **The Stretch:** Very slowly, begin to straighten your legs. As you do, concentrate on keeping your thighs against your chest. Take as much time as you want in your progress toward straightening your legs.

    At some point—farther away from the floor if you need more flexibility work, closer if you are more flexible to begin with—your chest will come away from your thighs. This is okay. Continue your slow descent toward the floor. When your legs become so straight that you have to release your arms from behind your legs, gently place your arms by your sides without disturbing your position.

    Stay in your final position a bit longer, reaching for the feeling of new length in your lower back and sacrum. This stretch works well when you perform it twice.

- **Enhance Your Flexibility:**
  The special character
  of this stretch will allow
  you to explore the feeling
  of length in your lower
  back and sacrum. Many
  stretches exist for this
  general area, but to make
  them effective you must
  first discover how to feel
  length in the area. Take
  your time with the stretch
  and let your body figure
  out this new feeling.
  It is an important key to
  attaining a flexible back.

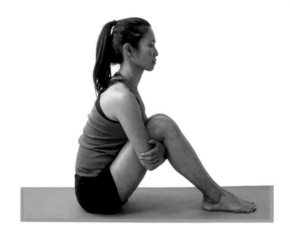

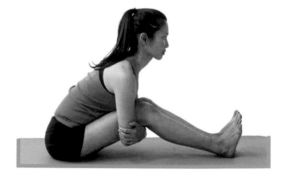

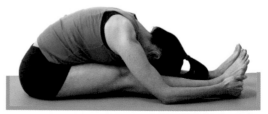

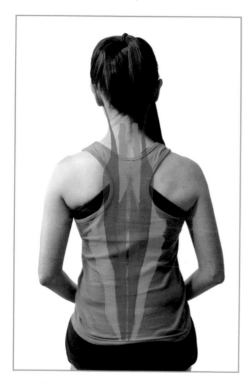

Note: See above for the muscles stretched and opposite for how to do the stretch.

ENLIST YOUR MIND

Keep thinking: lift up, up and forward, up and forward. Be patient with your mind–body connection. If you discover that when you gave the signal to lengthen your lower back, you have cricked your neck instead, then you know your body computer does not yet have a program for the thought you are sending it. Take a breath. Start again; repeat the signal. Leave it for the day; try it again the next day. You are educating your body to interpret the signals your mind sends it. You may be surprised at how much your body learned the next time you try this.

KEY TO MUSCLES
Erector spinae:
Iliocostalis
Longissimus
Spinalis thoracis

Multifidi

5 lower back (extension): chest and pelvic lift

- **The Setup:** Lie on your back on the floor, using a carpet or a mat for comfort. Bend your knees and place both feet on the floor. Place your arms by your sides. Open your feet wider than your knees, and test the range by pressing your knees inwards. If your knees touch, open your feet a bit wider. When you go into the stretch and bring your knees together, you want to be able to get to the end of your knees' range without having them touch each other.

- **The Stretch:** Lift your chest up onto your shoulders. You may have to adjust your shoulders a bit forward or toward each other, to make sure your chest is well supported. Make sure your neck remains relaxed. You should be resting your lifted chest on your shoulders. Then, lift your sacrum and low spine up into the air. Lift as high as you can; then bring your knees together at the height of the stretch.

  In this stretch, you are creating a beautiful spinal-extension arc in your back. Reach for the feeling of stretch all along your back—from upper back to sacrum. Bringing your knees together will also create a widening stretch across your sacrum and lower back. Last, as you lift your sacrum toward the ceiling, look for stretch in your hip-flexor area—just where your hips crease in front.

- **Enhance Your Flexibility:** Keep any strain away from your lower back by concentrating on lifting the chest and the sacrum at the same time. Experiment with the different parts of this stretch gently. There are several different stretches happening here. This may be new territory for you, so you may feel sore in unaccustomed places the day after trying this technique.

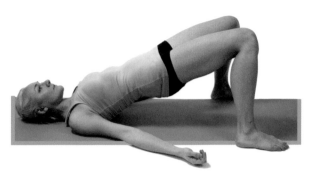

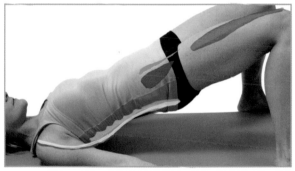

Note: In the illustration shown here, some of the back muscles being stretched overlay the arm. All muscles shown are stretching on both sides of the body.

6 lower back (extension): sacrum lift, kneeling

- **The Setup:** Kneel on the floor, using a carpet or mat if needed. When you execute any stretch, your body should feel comfortable. Tuck your toes. Place your hands behind you at sacrum/lower-back level.

  Here's the tricky part. Your palms should be facing your body, with the fingertips lifting the sacrum up and out of the pelvis. You might get into this position (which does feel strange at first) by starting with your hands by your sides with the palms facing back. Lift your fingers up so that your wrists extend, and move your hands behind your back, allowing your fingers to touch your spine. They should land in the area of the sacrum/lower back.

- **The Stretch:** Allow your fingers to give you the feeling of sacrum/lower-back lift, as you send them gently upward. Let your shoulders drop down and back and your chest lift as you feel your back lengthen into extension. Your neck follows the curve of the rest of your back. This stretch lends itself particularly to the breathing rhythm of exhale/lift the fingers, inhale/relax the finger lift. You can also press upward and hold in a gentle static stretch. Expect to feel some stretch in the hip-flexor area as well, where your hips crease in front.

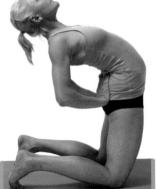

- **Enhance Your Flexibility:** Become aware of the degree of curve made by your entire spine.

Your neck (cervical spine) is part of that curve. It should curve only as much as the rest of your spine is capable of doing, and no more. Most people's neck curves have greater range than their back curves. A common mistake is thinking that you are curving your spine more by cricking your neck. This will just strain your neck, potentially causing problems with it. Instead, work on developing an accurate sense of the curve of your whole back. From this initial awareness you can progress to greater back extension range.

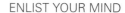

ENLIST YOUR MIND

Always think "up and forward," not just "forward." This will keep your back lengthening through its many vertebrae. You will never be in any danger of compressing the vertebrae together.

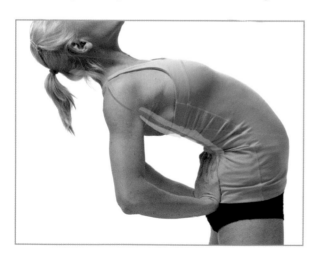

Note: On the artwork shown here, some of the back muscles being stretched overlay the shoulder and hand. All muscles shown are stretching on both sides of the body.

KEY TO MUSCLES
◻ Semispinalis capitis

Erector spinae:
◻ Iliocostalis
◼ Longissimus cervicis, thoracis
◻ Spinalis thoracis

7 lower back (extension): towel under pelvis

- **The Setup:** Lie comfortably on your back, with a carpet or a mat to cushion you, if you like. (To discourage ribcage arch, rest your arms by your sides.) Place a rolled-up towel under the curve of your lower back, just opposite your belly button.

- **The Stretch:** This is a stretch in which you can just relax and let gravity do the work. Once the towel is in place, allow your pelvis to relax into the floor below the towel, and your ribs to relax into the floor above the towel. Breathe deeply and regularly as you relax around your new lower-back curve. That's it. Just breathe and enjoy.

- **Enhance Your Flexibility:** The bigger the towel, the more your lower back will lift. If you have never experienced lower-back extension, this may be an unfamiliar feeling. In my own case, I was made so afraid of crunching my vertebrae together that I left lower-back extension out of my stretching repertory for a long time. Slowly get used to feeling a greater lower-back curve, and progress to a thicker towel roll as you learn to relax and let the curve happen.

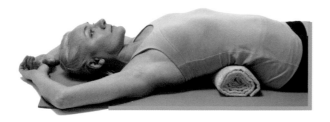

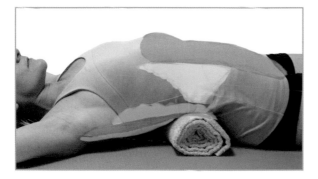

Note: All muscles shown are stretching on both sides of the body.

Here you have a chance to develop awareness both of your pelvis and your ribcage. If you have any sense of your ribs sticking up into the air, just keep talking to them and feel them against the floor when they let go. Your thought is: ribs and pelvis sink and relax.

KEY TO MUSCLES
Erector spinae:
▇ Iliocostalis
▇ Longissimus cervicis, thoracis
▇ Spinalis thoracis

▇ Rectus abdominis
▇ External oblique

8 upper back (flexion): crossed-elbows hug

- **The Setup:** Stand with your feet comfortably apart, about the width of your shoulders. Keep your knees slightly bent throughout the stretch. As you move into the stretch position, let your neck relax and your gaze drop.

- **The Stretch:** Cross your elbows at shoulder height. Reach your fingers as far around your shoulders as you can. If you can actually grab onto the inside edges of your shoulder blades, you will have a solid place to anchor your fingers.

Note: In the illustration shown here, some of the back muscles being stretched overlay the hand. All muscles shown are stretching on both sides of the body.

KEY TO MUSCLES
Rhomboids
Trapezius
Latissimus dorsi

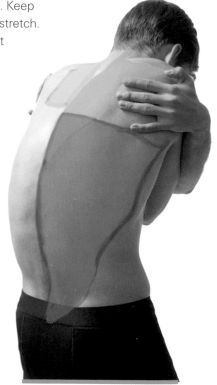

Slowly round your upper back and let it expand backward between your fingers. This is called "hollow back." To execute this position, you need a degree of body awareness. You must teach your body, in effect, how to do this hollowing. It is okay if you also feel your lower back rounding in response to the action of your upper back. You are just not concentrating the stretch there. Your pelvis can remain in neutral (neither tucked nor tilted) or slightly tucked. Just keep feeling for the stretch in your upper back.

- **Enhance Your Flexibility:** As your upper back widens in this stretch, you may be able to feel your shoulder blades actually separating a little, sliding outward along your ribcage. You can encourage this action with your fingers. You are not trying to pull the bones off your body— just to create a little more width in your back.

ENLIST YOUR MIND

Spare half a thought for your knees. Check that they have not crept up into the locked-out position. Keep them relaxed and slightly bent throughout.

9 upper back (flexion): backward pull, standing

- **The Setup:** Stand with your feet comfortably apart, about the width of your shoulders. Keep your knees slightly bent throughout the stretch. As you move into the stretch position, let your neck relax and your gaze drop.

  For this stretch, you will be leaning backward against a support that doesn't move. Some possibilities in your home may be (a) a doorway with mouldings on either side that extend out from the wall and form convenient finger holds; (b) a stationary floor-to-ceiling pole; or (c) two doorknobs on either side of an open door. Even a stretching partner holding the other end of a towel, as shown here, can work, if the person leans back and counters your pull.

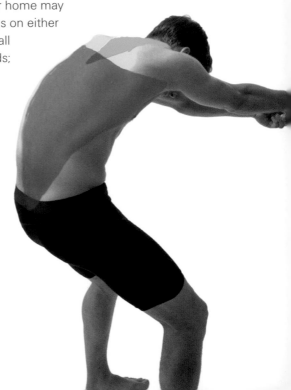

Note: All muscles shown are stretching on both sides of the body.

KEY TO MUSCLES
- Rhomboids
- Trapezius
- Latissimus dorsi

- **The Stretch:** Grasp your support firmly at approximately shoulder height, and slowly lean away from it, rounding your upper back and letting it expand backward. You are creating a "hollow back." To get in touch with the widening feeling of this stretch, just keep imagining that you can feel your upper back getting broader. You may need to try the position several times, perhaps on different days, to allow your body time to learn how to execute it well.

    This stretch is a more intense version of stretch 8, so you may want to try that one first. As in that stretch, don't be too concerned if you feel your lower back responding to your commands for your upper back. Just keep concentrating on what's happening in your upper back.

- **Enhance Your Flexibility:** Experiment with adjusting (a) your pelvis forward or backward a little; (b) your feet forward or backward a little; and (c) the height of your hands a little higher or lower. Concentrate on the stretchy feeling in your upper back, and how it is increased or diminished as you make these little adjustments. Discover the optimal stretch position for your body.

ENLIST YOUR MIND

Begin thinking about being able to tuck and tilt your pelvis. When you can do that, the next thing is being able to tuck and tilt your pelvis while keeping your ribs stationary. (See p. 34 for an introduction to these concepts.) Of course, these are movements for your body but the first step in your ability to do a movement is a clear understanding of what that movement is.

10 upper back (extension): towel under ribs

- **The Setup:** Lie comfortably on your back, with a carpet or a mat to cushion you, if you like. Your arms are resting by your sides. Place a rolled-up towel under your upper back, just at your chest line. For women, this will be your bra line; for men, the line of your nipples.

- **The Stretch:** This is another stretch using gravity to create upper-back extension length. All that is required is that you allow your ribs to relax below the spot where the towel rests. Slow, steady, deep breathing is your friend here. Increase to a thicker towel when your body adapts to the one you began with.

- **Enhance Your Flexibility:** The human back wants to expand—in every direction—simply because increased range feels good. As you practice this stretch and allow your back to get used to lengthening in extension, your back may thank you by letting you experience increased extension range. This is the opposite of a vicious cycle. You ask your body for length. It realizes you have its best interests in mind and complies with more length. And the next round—more flexibility.

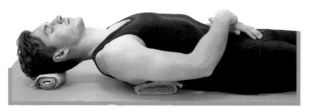

ENLIST YOUR MIND

Imagine your ribs and the tops of your shoulders melting, and sinking down to the floor on the upper and lower sides of the towel. Feel the small curve in your lower back, and send a quiet command to your pelvis to relax as well.

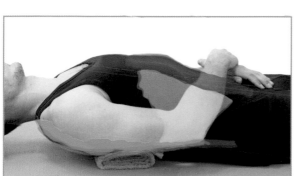

Note: In the illustration shown here, some of the back muscles being stretched overlay the arm. All muscles shown are stretching on both sides of the body.

KEY TO MUSCLES
Erector spinae:
█ Iliocostalis
█ Longissimus

█ Multifidi
█ Rectus abdominis
□ External oblique

11 upper back (extension): arms long, all fours

- **The Setup:** Get into the all-fours position on the floor. Your body is a table top: knees under butt, hands under shoulders.

- **The Stretch:** Keeping your butt over your knees, extend your arms forward. Sink your chest through your shoulders to create extension in your upper back. As you create more stretch in this area, you will be able to extend your arms farther forward, causing your butt to come forward of your knees. Check on your neck, making sure you are not thrusting your chin forward and causing a crick in your neck. Gaze downward, or along the line of the floor, to let your neck relax.

  You are working on developing the feeling of gently sinking your chest through your shoulders.

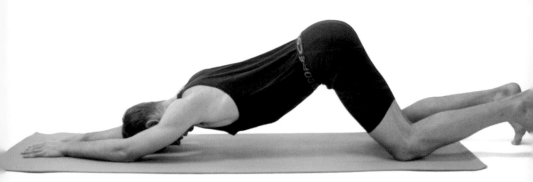

- **Enhance Your Flexibility:** The feeling of sinking your chest through your shoulders is an unfamiliar one for many people. The upper-back area is addressed less often in stretch routines. Since lower-back problems commonly abound, the average person will normally encounter those stretches more often. You may experience some soreness in this area when you first work on opening up your upper back. As long as you work gently, this should pass.

ENLIST YOUR MIND

This is a more intense version of stretch 10. It is a good idea to practice stretch 10 before proceeding to this stretch. Then carry the feeling of your upper back curving over the towel in your mind, and remind your body of that feeling when you practice this one.

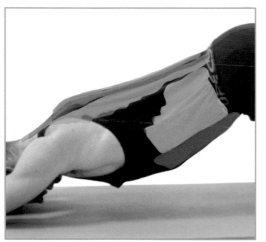

Note: All muscles shown are stretching on both sides of the body.

KEY TO MUSCLES
Erector spinae:
☐ Iliocostalis
■ Longissimus

☐ Multifidi
☐ External oblique
■ Rectus abdominis

12 full spine: extension (sphinx)

- **The Setup:** Lie on your stomach on the floor, using a mat or carpet for comfort. Begin with your arms extended in front of you, palms down. Lift your head slightly off the floor, with your neck long: you are gazing down at the floor. Your legs are long, with your feet stretching out behind you.

- **The Stretch:** Take a breath, and as you do, let your chest lift a little from the floor, making a slight upward curve with your neck and head. As you exhale, begin to move through an upper-body wave with the top of your head leading. Your head dips forward and comes up, followed slowly by your chin, your neck, your chest, your shoulders.

  As you create this wave, and your chest begins to lift off the floor, draw your straight arms back along the floor, creating a pull as your forearms head for their destination directly under your shoulders. Throughout the stretch duration, this gentle pull backward of the forearms continues.

  Once your forearms are in place under your shoulders, keep them there. The pull backward is isometric: your arms are not actually going to move, just exert pressure backward so your upper-back muscles will contract, creating traction and length all the way down your back. Enhance this feeling of back length by stretching your toes out behind you.

  Roll your shoulders down to lift your chest, and lift the back of your neck to create length. Slowly turn your head to the left. Feel how this adds extra length to your spine. Slowly return your head to the center. Repeat the head turn to the right.

- **Enhance Your Flexibility:** The main purpose of this stretch is to create extra space between the vertebrae of your spine. This will give you ease and freedom when you move, and make injury from sudden movements less likely. As you hold the stretch, continuing to create gentle spinal self-traction, look for an elusive sense of "well-being" when your sacral and lower-back vertebrae decompress. You may feel "relief" or "release"—or just surprise when you stand up and feel taller.

ENLIST YOUR MIND

Increase the effect of this stretch by picturing your spinal column and its vertebral discs. They are separated by a cushion of cerebrospinal fluid, which lubricates the joints and creates ease and fluidity in your movement. As you execute gentle self-traction, imagine those discs pulling slightly more apart, allowing more fluid in to cushion movement.

KEY TO MUSCLES
Erector spinae:
Iliocostalis
Longissimus

Multifidi
External oblique
Rectus abdominis

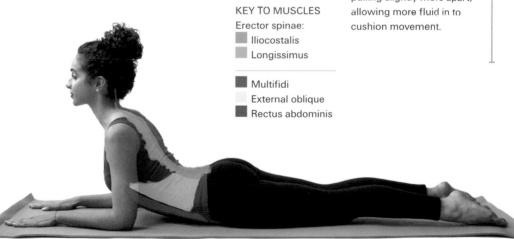

Note: In the illustration shown here, some of the muscles being stretched overlay the arm. All muscles shown are stretching on both sides of the body.

13 full spine: side, using chair

- **The Setup:** Sit on a stool or chair with your knees bent and feet on a stool rung or on the floor. Keep your shoulders facing forward; be sure you don't turn them to the side. Lift your left arm up at your side, palm facing inward. Grasp a stool or chair leg with your right hand. Look straight ahead. It may be helpful to check your position in a mirror.

- **The Stretch:** Begin to reach your long left arm slowly to the right. Counter the weight shift created by pressing your left sitting bone down onto the stool or chair. You will feel the stretch in your left side. As you lean farther to the right, you will

KEY TO MUSCLES
Erector spinae:
- Iliocostalis
- Longissimus

- Multifidi
- External oblique

be able to move your right hand farther down the stool or chair leg and feel more stretch. Try pulling upward with your right hand to see if that will increase your feeling of stretch. Your neck curve matches the curve of your arm. Repeat on the other side.

Your goal here is to feel the stretch along the left side of your torso. If you feel it in your arm instead, try settling your shoulder into its socket to relax your arm. It takes a little practice to master the feeling of a long arm that is reaching but not working. Instead the back supports it—in this case the side of the back.

• **Enhance Your Flexibility:** To get the right placement of your head relative to your arm, bring up your right arm to complete the oval shape begun by the left arm, and place your head exactly in the center of the two. When you return your right arm to its position on the stool or chair rung, your head should exactly match the curve of your left arm.

14a spiral: both knees to side, supine

Along with stretches 12 and 13, this group of three stretches addresses the full length of your spine. You may find 14a the gentlest. To add a little more intensity, experiment with 14b. The 14c position is not necessarily more intense or more advanced; rather, because you're sitting up and using your arms to help your body stretch, it requires more effort and is less relaxing.

- **The Setup:** Lie on your back on the floor, using a carpet or mat for comfort. Place your arms by your side, palms down, forming an "A" shape (fingers reaching away from you at 45 degrees to your torso).

- **The Stretch:** Bring both your knees as far in to your chest as you can. Drop both knees over to the left side and let them rest where they fall. Keep your right shoulder down on the floor. The stretch here is produced by your knees

KEY TO MUSCLES
- Gluteus maximus
- External oblique
- Iliocostalis
- Gluteus medius
- Longissimus

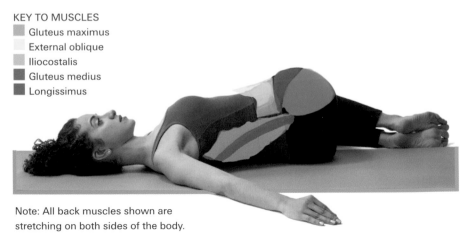

Note: All back muscles shown are stretching on both sides of the body.

pulling away from your shoulder, causing your spine to form its characteristic spiral shape. Repeat the stretch on the other side.

• **Enhance Your Flexibility:** This is the first stretch in this spiral series in terms of intensity. If your right knee is resting directly on top of your left knee, you have reached the maximum spiral stretch in this position. To add more intensity to your spiral, go on to stretches 14b and 14c.

If your right knee is hanging above the left one but not reaching it yet, that is okay. Any stretch requires practice, and learning things would be no fun if everything worked perfectly immediately. There will likely be a strong pull across your lower spine. If you can hold this pull without grimacing, allow the weight of your leg to bring your knee down gradually until, with enough familiarity with this stretch, your body is able to rest the right knee on top of the left. If the pull feels too strong at the moment, just place your left hand under your right knee. Give the knee as much support as it needs, so that you still feel a strong pull across your back, but not so much that you can think of nothing else.

ENLIST YOUR MIND

There will be some stretches you can do easily, and some that will challenge you and show you where your overall flexibility needs more work. This is true even for the most accomplished and advanced flexibility practitioner. Stretching is a life-long journey. Try on the thought that the stretches you come to love the most may be those that contributed most to your learning experience—the ones that initially were a struggle.

14b spiral: knee crossed over body, supine

- **The Setup:** Lie on your back on the floor, using a carpet or mat for comfort. Place your arms by your sides, palms down, forming an "A" shape (fingers reaching away from you at 45 degrees to your torso).

- **The Stretch:** Bring your right knee in to your chest as far as you can. Keep your left leg straight and in line with your hips: be careful that the left leg does not creep out more to the left. Cross your right knee over your body and let it fall to the left. You will feel the stretch diagonally across your back, especially in your lower spine. Make sure your foot is not resting on your leg. Repeat the stretch on the other side.

- **Enhance Your Flexibility:** Your right knee may touch the floor, or it may be suspended above it. Again, as in stretch 14a, use your left hand to give the right knee the support it may need, depending on the intensity of the pull across your back.

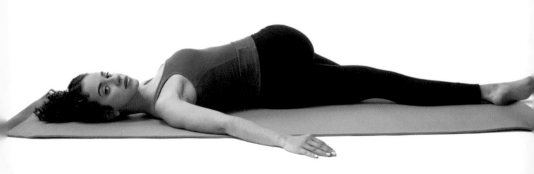

ENLIST YOUR MIND

In flexibility training, you will always be dealing with degrees of intensity in the stretchy feeling. That feeling will always be with you, even when you have a perfect 180-degree side split. It is the characteristic feeling you get when muscles stretch. When you are deciding how intense to let the stretchy feeling become, consider your body's comfort.

You and your body are in partnership in your flexibility training adventure. Bodies are very smart, and they don't like feeling pain. A body will always move away from pain—it's hard-wired that way to survive. Your body will be more likely to join your mind in achieving a common flexibility goal if you succeed in making stretching enjoyable for it. Just like your mind, if stretching is something your body likes and looks forward to doing, it is more likely to seek that experience, simply because it feels good. Of course, there is some crash-course training that takes stretching into the realm of pain, but I believe there are better ways to become flexible.

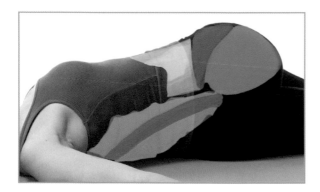

Note: Back muscles shown are stretching on both sides of the body.

KEY TO MUSCLES
- Gluteus maximus
- External oblique
- Iliocostalis
- Gluteus medius
- Longissimus

14c spiral: seated, using special arm positions

- **The Setup:** Sit on the floor, on a carpet or mat for comfort if you like. Stretch both legs out in front of you. Flex both feet; bend the right knee slightly, so that your right heel is about 6 in (15 cm) behind your left heel.

- **The Stretch:** Reach your left arm across your right knee. It will come to rest against your knee somewhere below your elbow. Your left arm will create one-half of the stretch. Place your right arm behind your back, right next to your spine. Rotate your fingers outward (backward) so that your shoulder

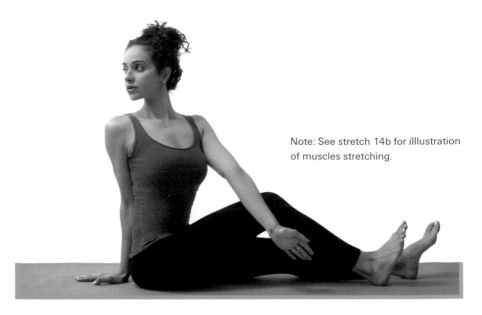

Note: See stretch 14b for illlustration of muscles stretching.

follows and rotates down and backward. This action allows your chest to lift as your shoulder drops. Your right arm will create the other half of the stretch. Finally, look over your right shoulder.

Press your right knee with your left arm, and press your right hand to the floor. Your shoulders will turn; your chest will lift as you drop the right shoulder; and you will look like the figures in an Egyptian painting—torso facing front, head in profile. Look for the stretchy feeling anywhere from lowest to highest point in your spine. It will show up in the spots where your spine needs most flexibility. Repeat the stretch on the other side.

• **Enhance Your Flexibility:** Crucial to the success of this stretch is the position of your right arm: right up against your back. This prevents any possibility of your leaning back. You are embracing your spine between your two arms and using your own body as the leverage to create the stretch. It may seem paradoxical as you sit in this upright position, but your spine can actually learn to relax and rest even when it lifts, as your two arms twine around it.

ENLIST YOUR MIND

Here you are always thinking: back lifts up and around; chest lifts up; shoulders drop. A good image for your brain is the barbershop pole, whose stripes spiral endlessly upward. That's what your spine does in this position. Keep thinking how it turns, how all the little muscles close to the spine enable it to spiral continuously up and up, as long as you hold the stretch. Your spine is a marvelous thing.

ABDOMINALS

When you want to eliminate back pain, stretching your abdominals is always a good place to start. Lengthening this area allows your diaphragm more movement, which frees your breathing. Plus, your stomach is directly opposite your back. As you lengthen both areas, you create more space between each vertebra, increasing your cerebrospinal fluid cushion.

In this section we will cover stretches for the major abdominal muscles—which pull the spine into flexion, rotate the torso, and support it. The two stretches described here address all the relevant abdominal muscles. Abdominals also stretch in: lower-back extension—stretches 5–7; upper-back extension—stretches 10–11; and full spine—stretches 12–14.

Causes of stiff, sore, or aching abdominal muscles/muscles in spasm

Injuries eased by stretching

Additional uses

- Using your abdominal muscles to support your torso in an awkward position—such as reaching underneath a sink or bathtub to clean the area. This is a case of sustained muscular effort: you must hold yourself in the position long enough to get the area clean.
- Strenuous or unaccustomed physical activity—such as your first attempts at doing pull-ups. Although pull-ups primarily involve back strength, the abdominals are heavily engaged, and the resulting post-exercise soreness may take you by surprise.
- Playing sports or doing activities that require a lot of core engagement—basketball, golf, running, walking, chopping wood.
- Playing sports or doing activities that require a lot of torso rotation—golf, racquetball/handball, throwing sports, chopping wood.

· ·

- Abdominal muscle strain.
- Hip-flexor strain.
- Iliopsoas (hip-flexor) tendonitis.

· ·

- Before and after playing sports requiring extensive core engagement or torso rotation—basketball, golf, racquetball/handball, running, throwing sports, walking.
- To relieve stiff back muscles: doing abdominal stretches may also help with back soreness.

Pinpoint the area of discomfort (this connects your mind with your body), and choose the stretch that most closely reaches that spot. **For guidance on stretch duration, see p. 25. To discover how to use breathing to deepen the stretch, see pp. 28–31.**

15 abdominals: finger-and-toe reach, supine

- **The Setup:** Lie on your back on a comfortable floor, complete with carpet or mat if you like. Stretch your legs out long, and your arms overhead, letting them extend along the floor behind your head.

- **The Stretch:** Point your toes and reach them away from your torso as far as you can. Feel your legs get longer. Reach your fingers along the floor behind you, allowing your arms to get longer as well. You will feel the stretch in the abdominal space between legs and arms. The space will elongate and hollow out.

  This stretch lends itself to a slow, inhale/exhale breathing rhythm. Inhale: gather yourself for the stretch. Exhale: reach your upper and lower limbs away from each other. Make each breath a long, deliberate one.

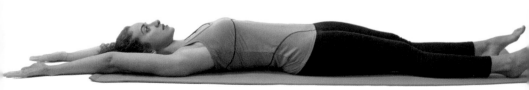

- **Enhance Your Flexibility:** Experiment with variations on this stretch. Stretch your right hand and right leg away from each other, while the left side relaxes. Feel how much longer your right side becomes. Then do the same on the left side. Also try reaching the right hand and left leg away from each other, to create a diagonal stretch feeling across your abdominal area.

Note: All muscles shown are stretching on both sides of the body.

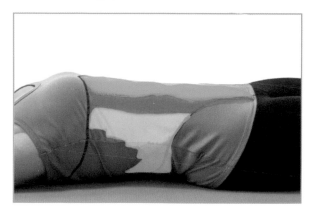

ENLIST YOUR MIND

Imagine that your toes are starting a chain reaction of length in your legs, and that your pelvis follows the legs away from your torso, creating extra space in your abdominal cavity. Likewise, think of your fingers starting the same chain reaction of length all along your arms down to your shoulders. Create abdominal space from above by allowing your shoulders to lift away from your ribs.

KEY TO MUSCLES
External oblique
Rectus abdominis
Transversus abdominis

16 abdominals: torso lift from floor, using arms

- **The Setup:** Lie on the floor on your stomach. Place your hands, palms down, under your shoulders.

- **The Stretch:** Slowly push your hands against the floor, gradually straightening your arms. This stretch also requires an ability to extend the low spine. If you feel mostly the low spine and not the abdominals stretching, practice stretches 5–7 and 12 first. Then come back to this one and see if you can locate the abdominal stretch feeling.

- **Enhance Your Flexibility:** You may need several repetitions of this stretch during a session before you can straighten your arms all the way. This is okay. Take as much time as you need to reach the full stretch. You may also build up to full range over several days or a week of practice.

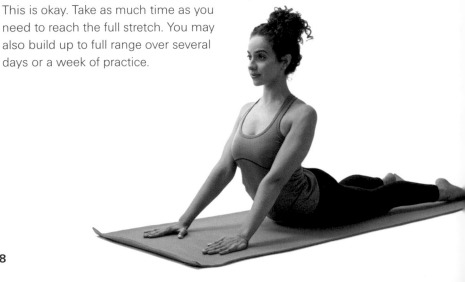

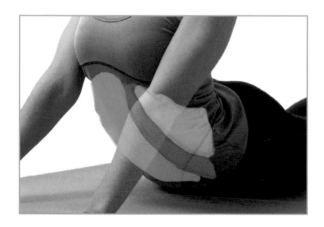

Develop your thought path: shoulders rolling down and relaxing back. Pubic bone sinking toward the floor. Those two points—shoulders and pubic bone—drawing away from each other create length up the front of your torso. Neck rises long out of the shoulders as they sink.

KEY TO MUSCLES
■ Rectus abdominis
■ Transversus abdominis
□ External oblique

Note: In the illustration shown here, some of the abdominal muscles being stretched overlay the arm. All muscles shown are stretching on both sides of the body.

HIPS

Because they are so close to it, flexible hips will go a long way toward easing your back. If the pain is severe, a good treatment tactic is working gently with the areas proximal to it—not directly at the site. Circuitous treatment is often effective: it relieves tension and muscle spasm all around the painful area. Hip stiffness can also contribute to creating pain, as when habitually tight hip flexors induce an overworked lower back.

In this section we will cover stretches for the hip flexors, the buttocks, and the side hip. The side-hip stretches—less commonly done— are particularly worth including in your quest for freely moving hips. Add to this group the inner thighs from the Thighs section (see p. 100), and you have a complete hip-opening sequence.

Causes of stiff, sore, or aching hip muscles/ muscles in spasm

. . . .

Injuries eased by stretching

. . . .

Additional uses

Pinpoint the area of discomfort (this connects your mind with your body), and choose the stretch that most closely reaches that spot.
For guidance on stretch duration, see p. 25.
To discover how to use breathing to deepen the stretch, see pp. 28–31.

- Running or hiking along steep inclines or declines.
- Sitting at a desk all day (or other long sitting session).

....

- Lower-back muscle strain.
- Lower-back ligament sprain (mild).
- Piriformis syndrome.
- Snapping hip syndrome (sometimes caused when your butt muscle "clicks" over your thigh bone).

....

- Before and after playing sports that use the hips a lot—such as cycling, golf, running, walking.
- To protect your lumbar curve. If the external hip-rotator muscles become tight, they pull on the lower back and the lumbar curve flattens. Without their natural curve, your lumbar discs are more likely to be compressed when you maintain a standing position. If you play sports, this problem is compounded.
- To release tight "turnout" muscles. Although this book does not cover stretches for dancing, many people—especially women—studied classical ballet for a time as children. If you have this training, take a look at the habitual rotation of your leg, starting up at your hip. If your toes are positioned outside your heels, and this feels natural, you may have tight external hip rotators (the muscles that rotate your hip and toes out) and not realize it. Or, do you walk with "duck feet"? Stretch these muscles with stretches 20–22. (Stretching the external hip rotators and strengthening the internal hip rotators—the muscles that rotate your hip and toes in—will give you balance between the muscle groups.)

17 hip flexors: knee-to-chest pull, supine

The following three stretches are a progression from least intense to most intense. If you are in pain or just beginning your flexibility training, experiment with stretch 17 first. When your body gets familiar with feeling the hip flexors stretching, you can add stretch 18, and finally stretch 19. Use the feeling in your body as your guide to how much stretch you can achieve on a particular day.

- **The Setup:** Lie on your back on a comfortable, supportive surface, with your legs at full length. Lace your fingers around your bent left knee and pull it to your chest, keeping the right leg straight. (You also have the option to pull behind your thigh, if pulling the knee feels uncomfortable.) Check your pelvis position. Make sure it is even—meaning that one pelvic bone is not lifted more toward the ceiling than the other, or more toward your shoulder than the other.

- **The Stretch:** Press your straight right leg to the floor while hugging your bent left knee to your chest. You will feel the stretch in the front of your right hip—where your hip bends when you lift your knee. Either hold the maximum position or gently press/pull and release in a slow rhythm (see Breathing, p. 28). Repeat with a straight left leg and bent right knee.

- **Enhance Your Flexibility:** Stretch and point your toes. Make your straight leg even longer by sending your thigh and calf away from your torso. Your whole leg will come alive with vitality, creating more space in the front of the hip.

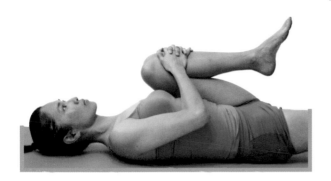

ENLIST YOUR MIND

Keep the back of your neck long—make sure your chin does not stick up toward the ceiling. Develop a strong mental connection with your body by gently reminding yourself to lengthen your neck. Soon you will find that your neck lengthens automatically.

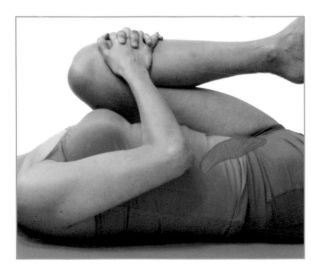

KEY TO MUSCLES
■ Iliopsoas (psoas major and minor, iliacus)

hips **83**

18 hip flexors: lunge, standing

- **The Setup:** Stand with your right leg forward and left leg behind you. Adjust the width of your stance for balance: if you need more stability, stand with your legs a little more apart. Toes should line up in front of heels—make sure they are not rotated outside your heels. Your front knee can be a little behind the ankle—just not in front of it. This protects your knee from strain. Hold your neck in a comfortable position—neither too lifted at the chin nor too bowed toward your chest. Just comfortable, without strain. Looking straight ahead helps to accomplish this.

  Your pelvic position is important here. Make sure your hip bones are even—top to bottom and front to back. (See "Enlist Your Mind," right.)

- **The Stretch:** Gently tuck your pelvis. The stretch will appear in the straight left leg—the back leg—at the hip-flexor level in front. At the same time, sense what's happening with your back leg: keep it straight. You can think: heel down, pelvis tucked. Repeat with right leg behind and straight, and left leg in front and bent.

- **Enhance Your Flexibility:** Experiment with what you feel when you send your front knee a little more forward toward your toes—a little more knee bend, then a little less. Just make sure your knee does not pass forward beyond your ankle.

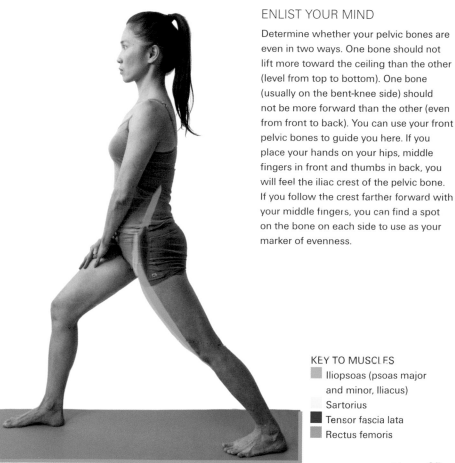

ENLIST YOUR MIND

Determine whether your pelvic bones are even in two ways. One bone should not lift more toward the ceiling than the other (level from top to bottom). One bone (usually on the bent-knee side) should not be more forward than the other (even from front to back). You can use your front pelvic bones to guide you here. If you place your hands on your hips, middle fingers in front and thumbs in back, you will feel the iliac crest of the pelvic bone. If you follow the crest farther forward with your middle fingers, you can find a spot on the bone on each side to use as your marker of evenness.

KEY TO MUSCLES
■ Iliopsoas (psoas major and minor, Iliacus)
□ Sartorius
■ Tensor fascia lata
■ Rectus femoris

19 hip flexors: lunge, kneeling

- **The Setup:** Kneel with your right leg forward and left leg behind you. Adjust the width of your stance for balance: for more stability, move your forward leg a little farther to the right. Your right toes should line up in front of your heel—make sure they are not rotated outside your heel. Your front knee can be a little behind the ankle—just not in front of it. This protects your knee from strain. For more support, kneel between two chairs, and place your hands on them if needed. Otherwise, place your hands lightly on your front thigh. Hold your neck in a comfortable position—neither too lifted at the chin nor too bowed toward your chest. Just comfortable, without strain. Looking straight ahead helps to accomplish this.

- **The Stretch:** Gently tuck your pelvis. The stretch will appear in the left leg—the back leg—at the hip-flexor level in front. When you experience the stretch in the right spot, you can intensify it by moving your front leg a little more forward. Ultimately, and with practice, your back hip will be much lower to the ground. On your way there, you will have moved your front foot forward in many small increments.

  Now comes an important point, which cannot be stressed enough. The hip-flexor stretch contains the beginning of a lovely back extension—also called an arch. Whenever we practice developing the back extension, we always encourage length: spine goes up as well as forward, to avoid scrunching the lower spinal vertebrae together. Repeat the stretch on the other side

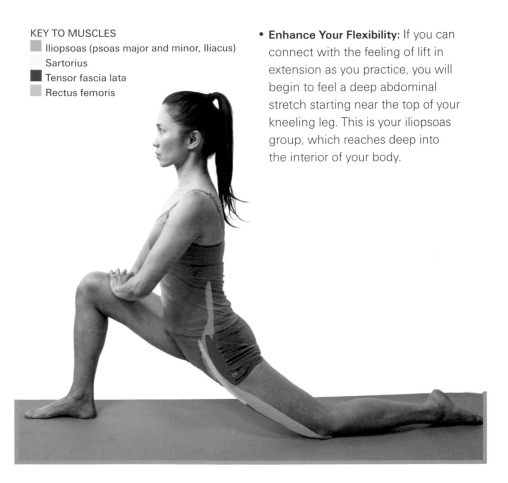

KEY TO MUSCLES
- Iliopsoas (psoas major and minor, Iliacus)
- Sartorius
- Tensor fascia lata
- Rectus femoris

- **Enhance Your Flexibility:** If you can connect with the feeling of lift in extension as you practice, you will begin to feel a deep abdominal stretch starting near the top of your kneeling leg. This is your iliopsoas group, which reaches deep into the interior of your body.

20 buttocks: ankle crossed over knee, seated

- **The Setup:** Sit on a supportive chair (not an armchair) with your right foot on the floor and your left ankle crossed over your right knee. Adjust your left ankle so that it feels comfortable—make sure the ankle bone isn't digging into your thigh. Open your left knee out to the side.

- **The Stretch:** Lifting up your sacrum (pelvis) and lower back out of your hips, begin to lean slowly forward, keeping your back flat. The stretch will appear in the left side of your butt. The feeling in the muscles you are targeting for this stretch should be immediately obvious. A steady exhale–stretch/inhale–relax rhythm is a good tactic for this stretch. Repeat the stretch on the other side.

- **Enhance Your Flexibility:** When you're ready for more intensity, lean steadily forward without relaxing on your inhale. Keep your back as flat as you can. These two actions will develop intensity. Your goal is touching your chest to your thighs. Although you may not get there for a while, if you practice you will notice your chest getting definitely lower.

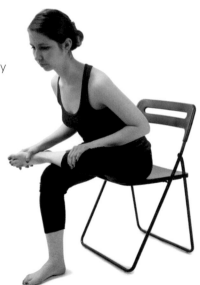

ENLIST YOUR MIND

On this one, your stretching mantra is: flat back, flat back. Think of lifting your pelvis up and away from the legs. Create lots of mental space in your hip joint, and soon there will be physical space there, making it easier to bring your torso up and forward.

KEY TO MUSCLFS
- Inferior gemellus
- Obturator internus
- Superior gemellus
- Gluteus maximus

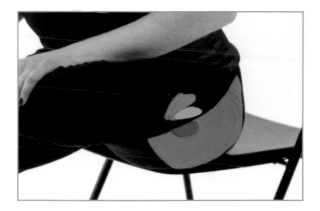

Note: The three deep hip-rotator muscles are actually located within the buttocks. For the purposes of illustration, we see them on the surface instead of deep inside and close to the pelvis.

21 buttocks: cross-body lower-leg lift, supine

- **The Setup:** Lie on your back on the floor, using a carpet or mat if you want some cushioning. Stretch your legs straight out. Bend your right knee, open it out to the side, and hold your right ankle with your left hand. This is similar to the setup position in stretch 20, except that you are holding your right foot in your left hand instead of resting it on your left knee. Reach your left hand over or under your ankle—whichever position feels more comfortable. Right hand rests on the right knee.

- **The Stretch:** At the same time, pull your right ankle toward your chest and push your right knee away from it. You are trying to bring your right ankle to a position directly across from your right knee. Optimum position for this stretch is lower leg parallel to shoulder- girdle line. Look for the stretch in the right side of your butt. Repeat the stretch on the other side.

- **Enhance Your Flexibility:** When you first practice this stretch, it may be very tempting for your head to lift off the ground because your outside hip is so tight. You can certainly start this way, supporting your neck flexors by gently pressing your tongue to the roof of your mouth. After you spend some time in this stretch, and your body figures out what you are asking it to do, you will find your head gently releasing to the floor. Keep your left leg as straight as you can while stretching the right side of your butt.

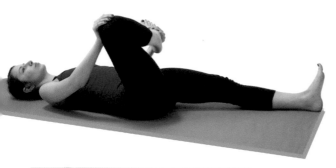

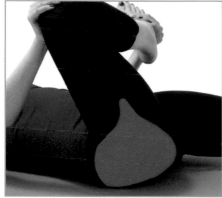

KEY TO MUSCLES
Gluteus maximus

ENLIST YOUR MIND

It is important to monitor the position of your neck. During the stage when you are working on settling your back to the floor, your neck will likewise lift. You don't want to introduce any extra tension or vertebrae scrunching in your neck, and one way to keep your neck relaxed while working on relaxing your back is to place a rolled-up towel behind your head, just opposite the bridge of your nose. Adjust the size of the towel depending on how far your neck lifts from the floor. Then check in with your mind: neck relaxes on the towel.

22 buttocks:
crossed-knees foot pull, lying on back

- **The Setup:** Lie on your back on the floor, using a carpet or mat if you want some cushioning. Bend your knees and put your feet on the floor. Cross your left knee over your right, resting your left thigh on your right. (This is exactly the same thing you would do if you were sitting upright and wanted to cross your legs.)

- **The Stretch:** Lift your crossed knees toward your chest. Your right foot will be sticking out to the left, your left foot to the right. Reach up with your hands and grasp the outsides of your feet—right hand takes the left foot; left hand takes the right. Pull your feet farther out to the sides, away from each other. Repeat the stretch on the other side.

- **Enhance Your Flexibility:** This stretch sounds simple, but it requires more outside-hip flexibility than stretch 20, for example. You may want to prepare yourself with stretch 20 for a while before attempting this one.

  When you first get into this stretch position, you will feel a strong pull in the two sides of your butt. Your feet will not want to open, and your back may come off the floor. Your first task is to allow your back to sink back onto the floor—even before you increase the pull on your feet.

  Once you can sink your back to the floor, you can exert a little more pressure on your feet. You will gradually be able to move your hands from a position near your ankles to one farther along your feet toward your toes.

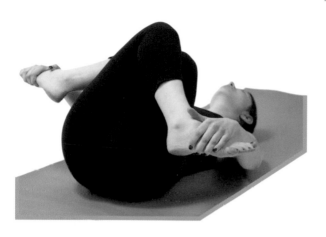

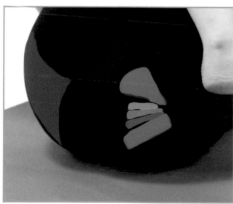

KEY TO MUSCLES
- ■ Gluteus maximus
- ■ Obturator externus
- ■ Superior gemellus
- ■ Obturator internus
- ■ Inferior gemellus
- ■ Quadratus femoris

Note: All muscles shown are stretching on both sides of the body.

23 side hip: knee push, lying on back

- **The Setup:** Lie on your back on the floor, using a carpet or mat to make you comfortable. Bend your knees and put your feet on the floor. Open your feet wider than your knees. Your knees remain in line with your hips, even though your feet are open.

- **The Stretch:** Drop your right knee inward, toward the floor. You should immediately feel a band of stretch around the outside of your right hip, beginning in your butt area and moving around to the side of your hip. Now cross your left knee over your right, and use the left knee to push the right gently toward the floor. Repeat the stretch on the other side.

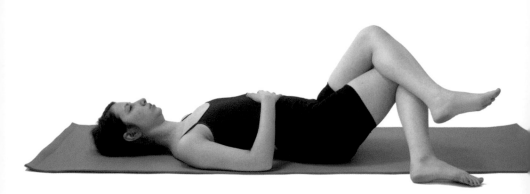

- **Enhance Your Flexibility:** Stretching the side-hip area is not done as often as, for example, quadriceps and hamstrings, so it is likely that this stretch will be unfamiliar to your body. The main action here is allowing the knee to relax toward the floor, adjusting the pressure of the assisting leg as necessary. Whenever you feel the tightness in your right hip release a little, increasing the pressure from the assisting knee will increase your range of motion in this area.

ENLIST YOUR MIND

Here your work is primarily calming your mind's unease, since this stretch is both powerful and most likely new territory for your body. Sometimes a panicky feeling can arise with a powerful stretch, a feeling of "what if I break in half?!" Slow, deep breaths will help your body find a resting place within the discomfort of the stretch.

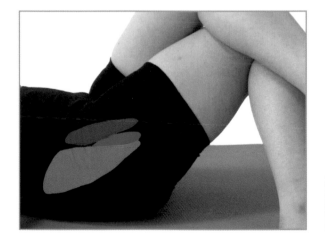

KEY TO MUSCLES
Tensor fascia lata
Gluteus minimus
Gluteus medius

24 side hip: towel under hip, lying on side

- **The Setup:** Lie on your right side with your legs stretched out, one on top of the other. Place a rolled-up towel under your right hip. The placement of the towel is important: it goes between your pelvic bone (iliac crest) and your thigh bone (greater trochanter). Get familiar with both these bony landmarks on your side before you place the towel. You don't need to know anatomy: just feel the bones that come to the surface at your hip and thigh.

- **The Stretch:** The stretch appears in the side of your hip facing the ceiling. In other words, the towel lifts your bottom hip so you can experience greater range in the top hip. Gently brace yourself with the open palm of your left hand. You can rest your head either in your hand (elbow bent) or on your straight right arm. Repeat the stretch on the other side.

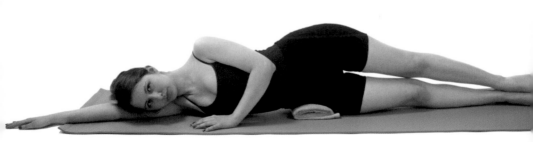

- **Enhance Your Flexibility:** For a greater stretch, use a larger towel. When you reach the point at which the world's largest towel still does not provide enough stretch because of the way it gives, try a rolled-up fitness mat or soft roller, which will elevate your hip higher. This is not necessary, however. At least at the beginning, the towel will work well.

ENLIST YOUR MIND

The trick here is to allow your abdominal and rib area to fall into the floor above the towel, and your thigh to relax into the floor below it. Keep sending thought messages of relaxation to those areas; allow them to drape over the towel and solidly settle onto the floor. Also, think left pelvic bone moving away from left thigh bone—and lots of space along the curve of your left hip.

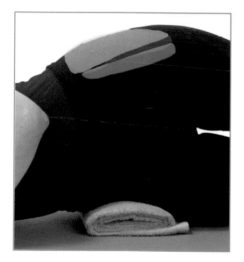

KEY TO MUSCLES
 Tensor fascia lata
 Gluteus minimus
 Gluteus medius

25 side hip: legs extending sideways, using arm

- **The Setup:** Lie on your right side at full length on the floor, using a mat or carpet to make you comfortable. Your legs are straight and stacked, one on top of the other. Lift your torso, keeping your head and shoulders in line with your legs and feet, and support yourself on your outstretched right arm. Make sure your right shoulder remains dropped and is not allowed to hike up.

- **The Stretch:** Gently push your right hip toward the floor. Without bending your arm, try to get the side of your hip flat against the floor. Of course, this won't happen, but a stretch will happen instead. In the photo you see the left foot crossed in front of the right leg, and the left knee bent. Experiment with this position to see if it helps you push your hip toward the floor more easily. Repeat the stretch on the other side.

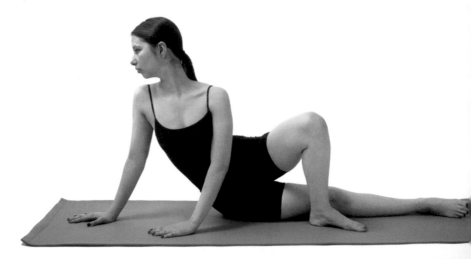

- **Enhance Your Flexibility:** Explore the balance between the distance of your hand from your body and your feeling of stretch. Adjusting the hand farther from or closer to your torso may enhance the feeling of stretch for you. This will be an individual adjustment for everyone.

  It is also important to keep your arm straight, but your shoulder dropped. This may take some practice. Many people have a tendency to bend the elbow when they try to drop the shoulder. You need the leverage that your straight arm will give you, but at the same time you must avoid sinking the neck into the shoulder.

ENLIST YOUR MIND

Connecting your mind to this stretch can be tricky. When you push your right hip toward the floor, at first you may feel your waistline stretching instead of the side of your hip. Be patient and keep working the hip gently toward the floor, searching for the feeling of stretch in a lower spot than the abdominals.

Note: In the illustration shown here, some of the muscles being stretched overlay the arm.

KEY TO MUSCLES
■ Quadratus lumborum
■ Tensor fascia lata
■ Gluteus medius

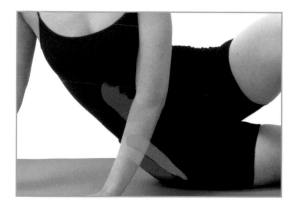

THIGHS

If you want convincing that stretching your thighs affects the condition of your back, just do the forward-bend test. Standing with feet under shoulders, roll down until your hands are as low as they will go. Note their distance from the floor. Then do a couple of hamstring stretches. Retest. This illustrates the famous lower-back/hamstring connection. If your back is especially painful, some gentle hamstring stretching is in order.

This section presents stretches for the inner thighs/groin, quadriceps, and hamstrings. To feel thorough, all-around hip opening, choose stretches for all three areas and do them in the same session.

Causes of stiff, sore, or aching thigh muscles/muscles in spasm

....

Injuries eased by stretching

....

Additional uses

- Playing sports or doing activities that use repetitive leg movements—such as basketball, cycling, running, walking.
- Any long sitting session—such as sitting at the computer or on an airplane flight.

- Hip-flexor strain.
- Iliopsoas tendonitis.
- Quadriceps strain.
- Quadriceps tendonitis.
- Patellofemoral pain syndrome.
- Patellar tendonitis.
- Lower-back muscle strain.
- Lower-back ligament sprain (mild).
- Hamstring strain.
- Piriformis syndrome.
- Groin strain.
- Tendonitis of the adductor muscles.

> *Pinpoint the area of discomfort (this connects your mind with your body), and choose the stretch that most closely reaches that spot.*
> **For guidance on stretch duration, see p. 25.**
> **To discover how to use breathing to deepen the stretch, see pp. 28–31.**

- Before and after playing sports or doing activities requiring constant thigh movement—such as basketball, cycling, running, walking.
- Before and after playing sports or doing activities requiring use of the inner thighs for side-to-side movement—such as racquetball/handball.
- To prevent hamstring tears in sports that require sprinting—such as racquetball/handball and running.
- To increase thigh range of motion, which helps create longer strides for a sprint.

26 inner thighs/groin:
knees over hips, supine

This sequence of three stretches for the short adductors involves bending and opening the knees. It begins with a less intense stretch that can serve as a warm-up for the others (stretch 26). The second stretch changes the angle between knees and hips, shifting the focus of the pull (stretch 27). The third stretch adds intensity by using the body's weight to stretch the inner-thigh muscles (stretch 28).

- **The Setup:** Lie on your back on a comfortable surface, using a mat or carpet to cushion your spine. Bend your knees, keeping them together and placing your feet on the floor. Bring your knees toward your chest, placing them in line with your hips.

    The line should be straight from your hips to your knees—perpendicular to the floor.

    Placing one hand on each knee, open your knees to the side. Relax your heels against your butt.

- **The Stretch:** Gently press your knees open with your hands. You will feel the stretch along your inner thighs between

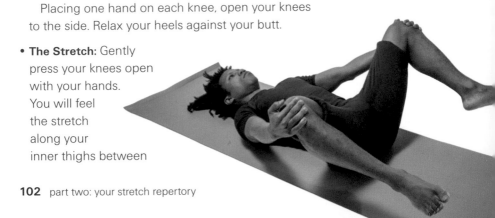

knee and hip. Hold the position for a static stretch, or use a gentle push-out-on-exhale/release-slightly-on-inhale technique.

- **Enhance Your Flexibility:** There will be a limit to how much you can increase this stretch using your hands to aid you. Press your knees down with more force—but still gently.

Note: All muscles shown are stretching on both sides of the body.

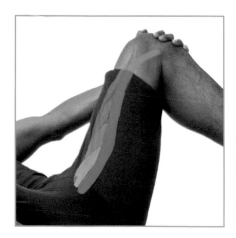

KEY TO MUSCLES
- Pectineus
- Adductor brevis
- Adductor longus
- Adductor magnus
- Gracilis

ENLIST YOUR MIND

This is a stretch that uses the trainer-assisted-stretch concept. When a trainer passively stretches your muscles, your only job is to relax those muscles, breathe calmly, and allow the trainer's pressure to deepen the stretch for you. Your hands, arms, shoulders, and back now become stand ins for the trainer. Make a separation in your mind between your upper body, which creates the stretch for you, and your inner thighs, which allow the stretch to happen. With practice, you will be able to relax some muscles and contract others.

27 inner thighs/groin: feet on wall, supine

- **The Setup:** Lie on your back on a comfortable surface, with a mat or carpet for support if you like, facing a wall. Bend your knees, with the soles of your feet together on the floor, right next to the wall. Crawl your feet up the wall and open your knees to the side. The outsides of your feet should now be touching the wall. Allow the outsides of your ankles to bend as you completely relax your feet against the wall.

- **The Stretch:** This is a passive stretch, which means you can let the position do the work for you while you concentrate on relaxing your muscles. Here the stretchy feeling is still in your inner thighs—but closer to your hip crease (groin) area. Keep breathing steadily and allowing your knees to continue to open.

- **Enhance Your Flexibility:** As you hold the position and your inner thighs relax and open more, try moving your body closer to the wall for a greater stretch. You will know the moment to do this, because the feeling of stretch recedes somewhat, allowing you to ask your body for more.

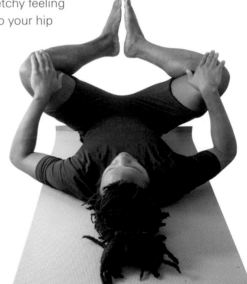

KEY TO MUSCLES
- Pectineus
- Adductor brevis
- Adductor longus
- Gracilis
- Adductor magnus

Note: In the illustration shown here, some of the leg muscles being stretched overlay the hand. All muscles shown are stretching on both sides of the body.

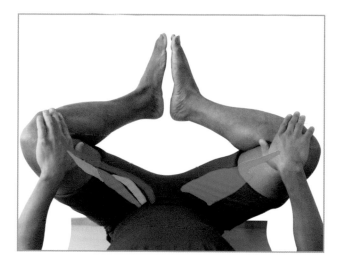

ENLIST YOUR MIND

This is a stretch in which your body is completely supported by the floor and the wall. You might try closing your eyes and imagining your knees opening wider. Pay attention to the feeling of stretch. As it gets less and you move your body closer to the wall, close your eyes again for a second round.

28 inner thighs/groin:
hips over knees, prone

- **The Setup:** Kneel on the floor in an all-fours position—pad the floor for comfort if you like. Begin to open your knees slowly out to the sides. Line up your knees directly under your hips. When your knees are open as far as they will go, place your forearms on the floor and get as comfortable as you can in the position. Make sure your knees are in line with your hips—neither in front of nor behind them.

- **The Stretch:** As soon as you start opening your knees, you will feel the stretch in your inner thighs.

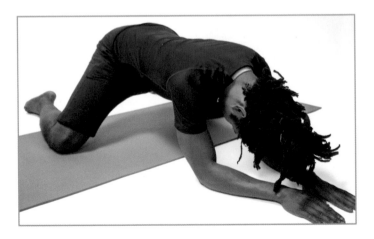

- **Enhance Your Flexibility:** This is the flip side of stretch 26, except that your weight is on top of the stretching muscles here, which makes this stretch more intense. Keep breathing regularly through the strong stretching feeling. You will be able to move your knees farther apart the longer you hold the stretch. Rock your butt a little behind your knees for a more intense feeling; then bring the knees back in line with your hips and see if you can move your knees farther apart.

ENLIST YOUR MIND

Imagine someone gently pressing on your sacrum/lower-back area, allowing your chest to come closer to the floor and your knees to separate more.

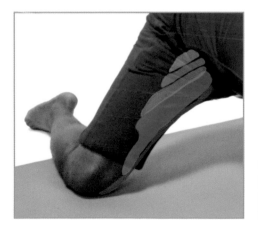

Note: All muscles shown are stretching on both sides of the body.

KEY TO MUSCLES

Pectineus
Adductor brevis
Adductor longus
Adductor magnus
Gracilis

29 inner thighs/groin:
side lunge, standing

In the next two stretches the legs are straight and open, allowing access to the long adductor muscles, and complementing stretches 26–28 for complete inner-thigh flexibility.

- **The Setup:** Stand with your legs open wide enough to fit your shoulders between your heels. Bend your left knee and shift your weight to the left side. Place your hands on your left knee for stability. Allow your torso to bend forward as you push into your left thigh with your hands. Your right leg remains straight, with the foot anchored in place. (Instead of placing your hands on your knee, you can hold onto a stationary support, for example, a doorway or post.)

- **The Stretch:** The stretch will appear on the inside of your right leg as you lean toward the left side. To protect your left knee from injury, it is important to keep it lined up with the left toes: make sure it doesn't roll inward. The placement of your right foot can be directly opposite or a little behind your left foot— whichever position you find more comfortable. Be careful not to move your foot too far backward, or the stretch will shift to your hip-flexor area. Keep the stretchy feeling in your inner thigh. Repeat the stretch on the other side.

- **Enhance Your Flexibility:** Once you locate the feeling of stretch along the inside of your right leg, you can increase that feeling by adjusting your degree of torso lean. Experiment with leaning a little more forward, a little more upright. You will also get a greater stretch by pushing your left hip more to the left side, allowing your right leg to move closer to the floor.

ENLIST YOUR MIND

Here you can experience the difference between an active and a passive stretch. Muscles in your left leg and hip are contracting, while muscles on the inside of your right leg are stretching. In this fairly simple stretch, with good strong support, your mind has a chance to sort out how it can pull off contracting and relaxing at the same time.

KEY TO MUSCLES
Pectineus
Adductor brevis
Adductor longus
Adductor magnus
Gracilis

30 inner thighs/groin: straddle against wall

- **The Setup:** Choose between bare feet or socks—whichever does not impede the further opening of your legs. Sit with the side of your torso next to a wall. Push your thigh and butt right up against it. Then turn onto your back and straighten your legs. Your butt and legs should end up right next to the wall and be supported by it.

- **The Stretch:** Slowly open your legs to the sides until you reach your maximum range of opening. You will feel a strong stretch in your inner thighs.

- **Enhance Your Flexibility:** Flex your feet, and activate both legs by lengthening through your heels. Now turn your toes a little toward the floor. This will rotate the muscles along the entire leg and produce a deeper stretch. Now breathe and relax your feet. Because of the comfortable lying position of your body, this is a stretch that lends itself to a static hold. Once your muscles get accustomed to how they feel in this position, you can stay in the stretch for two minutes, three minutes. Gradually increase the time.

  If your body really opened up for you, you must come out of the position slowly. If you shock your body, it may wish it hadn't opened. Try this method: place your hands one behind each thigh. Allowing your leg muscles to continue to relax, do all the work with your upper body. Pull behind the thighs so the knees bend a little. Push one leg over to meet the other (still without activating the leg muscles) as you roll over onto your side. Stay for a moment or so before you get up and move around.

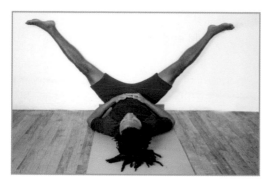

ENLIST YOUR MIND

This is a good stretch for closing your eyes, relaxing your legs as much as you can, and imagining your legs dropping more and more toward the floor. Then surprise yourself after your two-minute stretch and see how much closer to the floor they are.

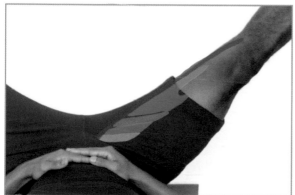

Note: All muscles shown are stretching on both sides of the body.

KEY TO MUSCLES
■ Gracilis
■ Pectineus
■ Adductor brevis
■ Adductor longus
■ Adductor magnus

thighs **111**

31 quadriceps: heel to buttocks, prone

- **The Setup:** Lie face down on the floor, with your legs at full length. The stretch will involve one leg and one hand, so you can either rest your chin on the other hand, or turn your head sideways and rest your cheek on your hand.

- **The Stretch:** Reach back with your right hand and grasp your right foot. Slowly bring your heel in toward your butt. The stretchy feeling will appear in the front of your right thigh (which is resting against the floor). Gently press your hip bone to the floor, taking away any bend in your hip. The right side of your body is now a straight line from shoulder to knee.

  When you first practice this stretch, you may be unable to reach your foot with your hand. You can hook a towel around your foot (either small or large, depending on the length you need) so that you can still pull your foot toward your butt. With practice you will gain more range, and the towel will become unnecessary. The stretch is at its maximum when your heel touches your butt. Repeat the stretch on the other side.

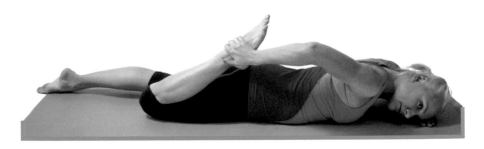

Make sure your legs are together. The knee of the stretching leg should be right next to the knee of the straight leg—not winging out to the side. Also, check that your foot comes straight toward the butt—not to the outside or inside of it. Correct alignment will make sure you have no joint problems as you practice.

- **Enhance Your Flexibility:** If you want a little extra flexibility challenge, adjust the position of your hand on your foot. Instead of placing it near your ankle, move your hand more toward your toes. This will add an extra dimension by also stretching the ankle and top of the foot.

ENLIST YOUR MIND

You can get a subtle increase of stretch in this position by feeling into the front of your thigh with your mind. Take a couple of breaths to eliminate mental distractions. Imagine that your thigh is getting longer because it is separating from the hip joint and creating more space there. As you think this, gently send your right knee away from your right hip along the floor. If you are really tuned in to your muscles, you can feel greater space in the hip joint and greater stretch in the thigh.

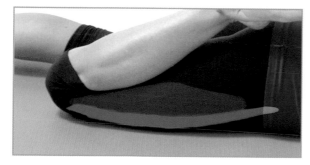

KEY TO MUSCLES
■ Vastus lateralis
■ Rectus femoris

32 quadriceps: back shin on wall, kneeling

- **The Setup:** Kneel on the floor in front of a wall—supported by a carpet or a mat, if you like. Place your left foot in front with your knee over your ankle. Place your right knee as close to the wall as you can, with your right shin resting on the wall. Either place your hands on your left knee for support, or hold onto a piece of furniture or a wall. Keep your torso upright, and your shoulders and neck relaxed.

- **The Stretch:** As soon as you place yourself in the setup position, you will likely start feeling this stretch in the front of your right thigh. This is a powerful move with the ability to increase your range of motion quickly. Consequently, the effort involved is considerable. Breathe. Relax into the position as much as you can. Repeat the stretch on the other side.

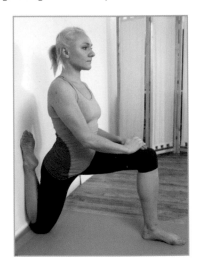

- **Enhance Your Flexibility:** You are already asking your body for a great deal of flexibility here. In comparison to this stretch, stretch 31 is much less intense. Another place you will notice stretch is up the front of your right foot, which is resting against the wall.

When you want to increase the stretching pull, gently tuck your pelvis and feel how the front-of-thigh stretch increases. Try a breathing rhythm: exhale/tuck your pelvis, inhale/release your pelvis.

ENLIST YOUR MIND

The stretch here is likely to feel extreme. This is not a position that requires you to find the stretch—it will be quite evident. Use your mind to quiet your feeling of panic. Keep breathing and reassuring your body inwardly that it is okay, that it is safe to open up. If you can remain in the position for as long as a minute, you will find your body already responding to your mental signals, quieting down, and settling into the stretch a little more.

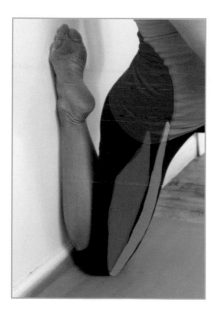

KEY TO MUSCLES
◼ Vastus lateralis
◼ Rectus femoris

33 hamstrings: one leg bent

- **The Setup:** Stand with your feet about shoulder-width apart. Bend your left knee slightly, and move your right foot out in front of the left to a comfortable distance. You should feel balanced. The position should be easy to hold. Flex your right (front) foot, and keep that leg straight. Your position is now: front leg straight, back leg bent.

   Place your palms on your right thigh, near your hip crease, and gently press. Make sure your pelvis is even.

- **The Stretch:** Keeping your back straight, begin to lower it slowly toward your thighs. You will feel the stretch in the back of the right (front) leg. Keep your neck curve in line with your spinal curve.

   Feel your way into this stretch. A long, slow pulse may work for you, or a static hold may be better. Once you become familiar with the position, you will be the best judge of what your body needs to allow it to expand its range of motion. There is some body weight leveraging the stretch; therefore, you can make this stretch more intense by leaning more weight forward. Always keep the back straight—"flat back" is the term used in fitness.

   Repeat the stretch with the left leg in front.

- **Enhance Your Flexibility:** What does an "even pelvis" mean? This term is often used, but perhaps not understood well. We want a level playing field from which to go into a stretch. You can locate your front pelvic bones just above your hip creases. When you perform this stretch, just make sure that the front pelvic bones are in line sideways. When someone does this stretch, it often happens that the straight front leg is allowed to pull the pelvic bone on that side forward. An even pelvis will always give you a better-aligned stretch.

ENLIST YOUR MIND

Keep thinking: neck in line with spine; neck is long. It is common for people to crick their necks in this stretch. This will cause imbalance to your cervical vertebrae if done habitually. We want to be in a more ideal position after performing stretches—not introduce more things to fix. Remember: your view is your legs, not what's in front of you.

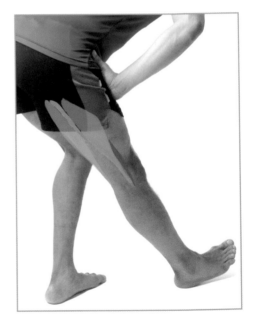

KEY TO MUSCLES
- Semitendinosus
- Semimembranosus
- Biceps femoris (long head)
- Biceps femoris (short head)

34 hamstrings: palms on floor, standing

- **The Setup:** Stand with your feet about shoulder-width apart and shoulders relaxed. With your knees bent, roll your spine slowly downward, beginning at the top of your head, tucking your chin, and slowly rolling down through all your spinal vertebrae. When you pass your waist with your head, pull in your belly button to support your lower back as you continue to descend toward the floor. Stop when you are at the full extent of your present hip-flexion range. Your head and neck remain relaxed. Your view is of your own legs. You may already be feeling a stretch. Note how far your fingers are from the floor, so that you can compare their distance after you execute the stretch.

ENLIST YOUR MIND

When you reach your current lowest point in this stretch, make sure your legs are straight and your neck is relaxed. Close your eyes for 30 seconds. Either count slowly to 30, or set a 30-second digital alarm to free your mind. When you open your eyes, you may be surprised to find how much closer to the floor your head and hands are. Perhaps in some unconscious recess of your brain, you don't believe you can place your palms on the floor. Use this mind trick to change that belief. Your range will increase, and you will feel better.

- **The Stretch:** Slowly straighten your legs. Take all the time you need. If you can straighten your legs without lifting your back up at the same time, you will achieve a deeper stretch. Here we emphasize stretch in the hamstrings. But keep in mind that, if your back is more in need of stretching, that is what you will feel. Any stretch that addresses the hamstrings will also lengthen the back. What you feel is determined by the area you most need to stretch.

- **Enhance Your Flexibility:** A variation of this stretch is to straighten first one leg and then the other, in a slow, alternating rhythm. Try the slow breathing rhythm: inhale/relax the knees; exhale/straighten one knee.

    As you allow one leg to relax when the knee bends, see if you can straighten the other leg without compensating by lifting your back. This will increase the stretch. Then try both legs together and see how much farther your fingers have progressed toward the floor.

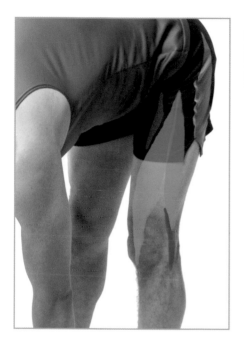

KEY TO MUSCLES
- ⬜ Biceps femoris (long head)
- ⬛ Biceps femoris (short head)
- ⬛ Semimembranosus
- ⬜ Semitendinosus

Note: The muscles illustrated are on the back of the leg but, for the purposes of illustration, are shown on the front of the leg. All muscles shown are stretching on both sides of the body.

35 hamstrings: leg on raised surface, standing

- **The Setup:** Stand on your left leg and lift your right leg onto a raised surface, such as a stool. To reach it more easily and get some extra support, slant your body relative to the stool. Move your left hip slightly left of the stool, allowing the right leg to rest slantwise on it. We are seeking even pelvic bones—side to side—to create the best angle for the stretch. So, when the right leg is up, check the pelvic-bone evenness. Locate your front pelvic bones by placing your hands on your hips, middle fingers in front and thumbs in back, to feel the iliac crest of the pelvic bone. Calculating your stance relative to your slantwise position, pull the right pelvic bone back so it is directly opposite the left one. Align your hips square to the direction you are facing—slantwise in this case. Now you're ready to stretch.

- **The Stretch:** As you lift your back straight up and away from your legs, lean slowly forward. Keep your back flat as long as you can. The stretch will develop in the back of your leg. When you can no longer keep your back straight and flat, allow it to curve forward, and bend to your fullest extent— today. Make sure your neck matches the curve of the rest of your spine, that is, keep your chin from jutting out. Repeat the stretch on the other side.

- **Enhance Your Flexibility:** On an exhale, flex your foot. As you inhale and relax it, try to bring your chest closer to your thighs. Repeat this inhale/exhale rhythm several times to increase your range. Another tactic is changing angles of the leg. Flex your foot and rotate your toes outward, away from the midline of your body. As you feel the increase in stretch in the back of your leg, try not to raise your back from its position. When you return the foot to its parallel position, see if you can lower your back still more. Spend some time coaxing more flexibility out of your leg.

ENLIST YOUR MIND

Keep developing your sense of lifting the back up and away from your legs. Visualize space in your hip joints to create this lift. Remember: your back is separate from your legs. It sounds obvious, but have you ever stopped to think that way when you are stretching? Try this concept and see how your stretch range improves.

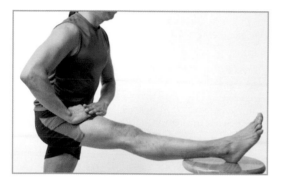

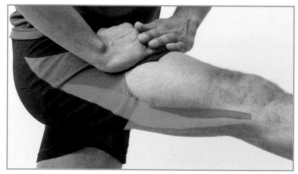

KEY TO MUSCLES
■ Biceps femoris (long head)
■ Biceps femoris (short head)

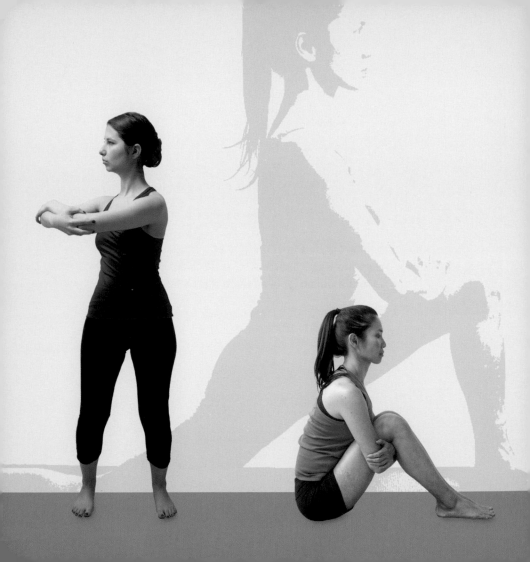

PART THREE:
STRETCH SEQUENCES

Discover recipes to make with your Part Two ingredient mix.
As well as learning how to warm up before stretching—and
finding out why warm-ups are important—you will find stretch
sequences to relieve areas of pain, increase range of motion,
and keep your body stretched throughout the day. There is
also advice on working out which muscles to stretch
according to the activity you want to do.

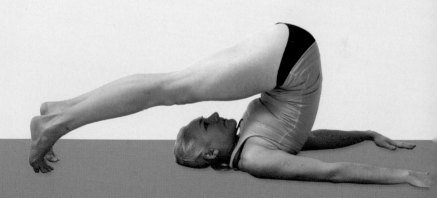

which muscles to stretch:
matching flexibility to activity

HOW TO CHOOSE

We know that flexibility is specific to each muscle group around a joint (see Introduction, p. 8). In fact, it is not only specific to each joint, but to each movement within a joint.

What does this mean? Take hamstring flexibility. When you stretch by standing on one leg and placing the other straight leg up on a surface (see stretch 35, p. 122), there are several ways to point your toes:

- Straight up toward the ceiling.
- Toward the midline of your body.
- Away from the midline of your body. (And variations in between.)

The range of motion in your hamstring (torso bent forward, leg straight) may not be equal in each of these toe positions.

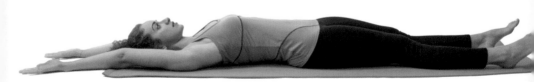

So, we all should stretch every muscle we can get our hands on, at every possible joint angle. On a regular basis. That would be the ideal thing. Hmmm.

I mention this to give you an idea of how large is the concept of having a flexible body.

Practically speaking, though, given the schedules of life, there may be some time limits on our flexibility sessions. So, here are some guidelines for efficient directions you can take as you pick muscles you want to concentrate on in your stretching practice.

First things first: definitely, everybody stretch your spine!

Attaining and maintaining a mobile spine is of paramount importance to your mobility. Your spine is an amazing, multi-movement structure, and you want to keep it that way. Because of the arrangement of its many bones, it has a large native repertory of movements: it can flex forward, extend upwards and back, extend laterally to both sides, and rotate to both sides. To a large extent, the condition of your spine determines your biological age (see Introduction, p. 8). Take a good look at people who are not able to bend and turn easily. The spinal stiffness you observe is largely what makes you perceive them as "old." Staying young—and being perceived that way—is largely a function of a "youthful" spine: flexible, easily movable without a second thought.

A good body-awareness goal is developing the feeling of each vertebra moving independently. Feel stretch all the way along your spine. When you do the Spinal Roll-Down and Roll-Up (see Moving Warm-Ups, p. 131), imagine each bone in the vertebral chain as a single pearl on a whole strand of them.

Two helpful techniques for creating this feeling are stretches 5 and 6 (see pp. 50 and 52).

For well-rounded spine flexibility, try out all the stretches in the Back section and see which ones help you most.

Clues elsewhere in this book

Many sections of this book necessarily dovetail and overlap. Look through all the sections of this part of the book (see pp. 124–165), and take an inventory of how your body feels, or think about what you're planning to do in the way of physical activity.

Stretch to relieve common areas of pain (see p. 144)
- Lower back and sacrum
- Hips

Note: When you want to relieve pain or stiffness, stretch not only in the area of actual soreness, but also look at areas distant from the site of discomfort. For example, stretching your upper back may eliminate lower-back discomfort.

Stretch to increase range of motion (see p. 152)
- Hamstring/lower-back connection
- Hip flexors/quadriceps

Stretch throughout your day (see p. 158)
- Upon waking in the morning
- Prolonged sitting
- Driving
- Before going to sleep

Remember, it is also important to stretch before and after common physical activities, such as cycling, running, sports (for example, basketball or swimming), walking, and yoga.

How much muscle range do you need?
Once you decide which muscles to stretch, think about what goal you want to set for their flexibility. What range do they need to have? As you have already read (see Introduction, p. 9), determine your flexibility goal according to the activity you want to be mobile enough to do. For example:

- **For daily life:** you need enough flexibility to bend down and pick up something you dropped on the floor.
- **For aerobic dance:** you need enough flexibility to lift your knee to 90 degrees without tucking your pelvis under.
- **For gymnastics:** you need enough flexibility to execute a split.

Figure out the range you need in a couple of ways:

- **For a life action, through your own observation:** to see over my shoulder, I must be able to turn my head a little farther.
- **For a new skill, from information given by a skilled instructor:** to execute a back bend well, my shoulders must be open enough to allow me to straighten my arms.

The flexibility reserve

In their book *Stretch to Win*, Ann and Chris Frederick speak about the "flexibility reserve." Through their experience working with many athletes, they have found that having 20 per cent more flexibility than you need for your activity makes injury much less likely. They help their clients develop this reserve in thew trunk, spine, shoulders, pelvis, and hips.

Extra flexibility helps you:

- If you fall and land in an awkward position. Your body tissues can handle being suddenly forced farther than their usual range.
- If you reach a little higher or farther back than normal in the heat of a game. You won't tear a muscle.
- In cold weather, when it's hard to keep your muscles warm. Your extra flexibility saves the day.*

* Ann and Chris Frederick, *Stretch to Win: Flexibility for Improved Speed, Power, and Agility* (Campain, IL: Human Kinetics, 2006), 180–81.

prepare to stretch: moving warm-ups

WHAT IS A WARM-UP—AND WHY DO IT?

The stand-alone flexibility training session is a "real" workout—although of a different kind. Therefore, warming up will help you to get the best results from a stretching session. The increase in core and muscle temperature provided by a warm-up makes stretching safer and more productive.

It is helpful to incorporate a series of stretches into your warm-up before a physical activity—like running, for example. But stretching is not a complete warm-up—it is a warm-up component.

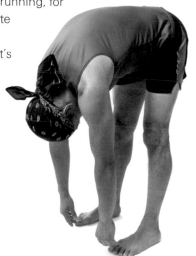

Just in case you are now confused, let's talk about what "warming up" before physical activity means. What should it accomplish? How does it justify the extra time it requires?

You warm up for two reasons: to prevent injury, and to prepare your body for optimum performance of a physical activity.

The warm-up accomplishes those goals by delivering the following benefits:

Group A
- Increases heart and respiratory rates, preparing your cardiovascular system for activity.
- Increases blood flow through your active muscles and hence delivery of oxygen and nutrients.
- Increases nerve impulse speed, making it easier to move your body.
- Allows muscles to contract and relax faster and more efficiently.

Group B
- Increases core and muscle temperature.
- Decreases resistance to muscle stretch-ability.
- Decreases muscle tension.
- Enhances connective tissue and muscle stretch-ability.

All the above benefits assist your body to work better, but Group A is especially helpful when you are proceeding from warm-up to sports activity, and Group B when you are focusing on increasing your range of motion through stretching.

So, what exactly do you do to warm up? Well, there are many opinions about it, but here are some guidelines:

- **First, if your chosen activity is a flexibility session,** doing five to ten minutes of some moderate-paced, general body movements will be enough to increase your body temperature. Getting warm enough to sweat is good—but getting tired during the warm-up is not. This is enough activity to prepare you for a productive stretching session—and that's what you get in this section.

- **Second, if your workout goal for the session is a more aerobically demanding physical activity**—such as running, cycling, etc.—stretch the muscle groups you will be targeting in your activity. You can accomplish this in about ten minutes.

- **Third, if you are on a team or practicing for an individual sporting event beyond the casual,** you may be doing some sport-specific drills as well, and finishing it all up with more stretching of the dynamic variety.

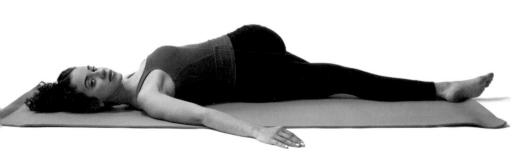

Some sports stretching experts advocate warming up for as much as 35 to 40 minutes before engaging in a sports activity. Obviously, if your entire workout time is 45 minutes or an hour, you will do a shorter warm-up.

The classic aerobic dance class always begins with an ideal warm-up:

1 Five minutes of big body movements, followed by

2 Five minutes of stretches in motion.

The beauty of (2) is that you are stretching, but you never stop moving. The warm-up prepares your body for the goal—nonstop movement for at least 45 minutes (exclusive of cool-down and ending stretch)—by warming up the core body temperature in (1) and by incorporating the appropriate stretches in (2). Perfect.

The upshot is: do you feel warm and ready to work? Dancers always say that their muscles work better in a warm room—that is, when your body and muscles feel warm, you're ready to go.

1 back

The two movements below—Spinal Roll-Down and Spinal Roll-Up—are meant to be performed one after the other without a pause.

In a class with an instructor guiding you, this would become obvious. But in a book, you necessarily have to read about the movements in sequence. Read the directions first, and then execute both movements smoothly.

As you get used to the movements, you can execute them a little faster. Instead of counting "eight" on the way down and on the way up, try counting a slow "four," letting your spine ripple as it moves.

ENLIST YOUR MIND

Spare half a thought for your knees: keep them generously bent. When we concentrate on a principal movement—such as rolling down the spinal vertebrae in sequence—we sometimes forget to check on what the rest of our body is doing. Bent knees: put this signal in the back of your mind. Thinking this helps to develop global body awareness.

1a spinal roll-down

- **The Setup:** Stand comfortably, with your feet as wide as your shoulders (not too narrow), your knees slightly bent, and your shoulders relaxed. Breathe easily and calmly.

- **The Movement:** Tuck your chin to your chest, and begin rolling your spine slowly down from the top of your head. Allow your extended arms to dangle freely, and your relaxed fingers to descend toward the floor. Feel each part of your body roll down in its turn. See if you can feel each separate bone in your back curving downward after the one above it.

When your head passes your waistline on its way down toward the floor, pull your belly button in toward your spine to protect the vertebrae of your lower back. Keep the back of your neck extended and relaxed. Your view should be your legs and feet—not what's in front of you.

Take a slow count of eight to roll down. Stop your roll when you reach your maximum downward range.

Perform three to five repetitions of the complete (a) Roll-Down and (b) Roll-Up sequence. Stop when you feel your spine start to become free and loose.

- **Enhance Your Experience:** You may want to start the downward movement using a big, exhaling sigh as you tuck your chin.

1b spinal roll-up

- **The Setup:** Perform this movement immediately after the Spinal Roll-Down. You will be standing with your spine bent as far down toward the floor as you can at this moment—without forcing. Your feet are as wide as your shoulders, your knees bent, your neck relaxed, your arms dangling.

- **The Movement:** Give your body the signal to roll up by pushing down into the floor slightly with your heels. At the same time, pull your belly button in to protect your spinal vertebrae as you curl them slowly up, one after the other. Your view is that of your legs and feet. Make sure not to look up—you will certainly crick your neck.

Take a slow count of eight to roll up. Feel your shoulders resettle themselves on your ribcage. The last thing to come up will be the top of your head.

Perform three to five repetitions of the complete
(a) Roll-Down and (b) Roll-Up sequence. Stop when
you feel your spine start to become free and loose.

- **Enhance Your Experience:** As you give the impulse
through your heels to start rolling up, you may
want to utilize an exhaling breath. As you roll up,
cultivate feeling each bone in your spine as it
regains its place on top of the one below it.

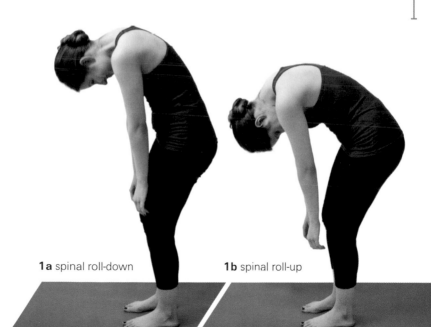

1a spinal roll-down   **1b** spinal roll-up

2 shoulders: arm circles

- **The Setup:** Stand comfortably, with your feet as wide as your shoulders (not too narrow), your knees slightly bent, and your shoulders relaxed. Breathe easily and calmly.

- **The Movement:** Swing one arm in a great arc, first forward, then up, then back, and around to your starting place again. Use momentum: as you begin your circle, it helps to bend your knees. Use the impulse you get from straightening them slightly to swing your hand at the end of your arm. The idea is to move only your shoulder—your wrist and elbow joints are relaxed, your fingers loose.

  Perform a set of eight circles front to back, then a set of eight circles back to front. Repeat with the other arm. When your shoulders start to feel loose, free, and warm, you are ready to go on to the next movement.

- **Enhance Your Experience:** To help you feel the essence of this movement, think of the great circle one end of a rope makes as you hold the other end anchored in your hand and swing it from there. Your hand is the free end of the rope. The impulse for the circle originates at the shoulder end of the movement. Your arm is dead weight—just like the other end of the rope.

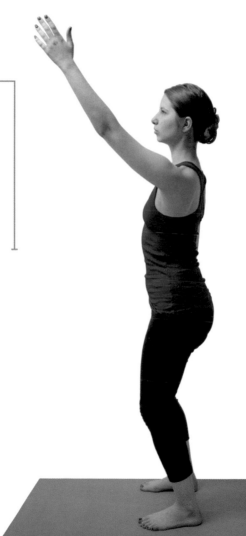

ENLIST YOUR MIND

Keep your neck relaxed and
your shoulders low as you
perform this movement.
When you move, you
always want to release
unwanted tension—not
create more of it.

3 abdominals:
side-to-side
"washing machine"

- **The Setup:** Stand comfortably, with your feet as wide as your shoulders (not too narrow), your knees slightly bent, and your shoulders relaxed. Breathe easily and calmly. Extend your elbows out in front of you, with each hand grasping the opposite elbow. Keep your elbows slightly lower than shoulder height, to avoid tensing up your shoulders. You are creating a firm upper-body structure, similar to what ballroom dancers do when they connect their upper bodies to form a stable "frame."

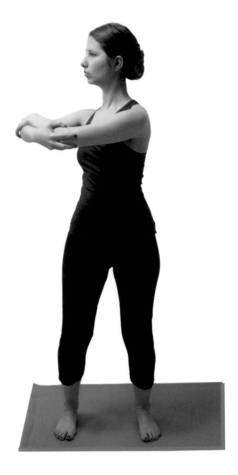

- **The Movement:** Keeping your hips facing straight ahead, turn the rest of your upper body—from the waist upward—first to one side, then to the other. Make this a continuous movement—side to side, side to side, with your whole upper body turning at once and your hips stable.

  The idea is to feel your abdominal muscles powering the turn for you. Everything else is stable and solid—upper and lower body both—and your abs are churning right and left, like a top-loading washing machine.

  To begin, perform two sets of eight repetitions (right and left is one repetition) at a fairly slow tempo. Then speed up slightly for two more sets, and slightly more again for the last two sets. This movement aims to get your core temperature up by engaging your abdominal muscles, and to access your deeper breathing.

- **Enhance Your Experience:** Turn your head in the same direction you turn your arms, looking over the midpoint of your forearms as you move. Focus to left or right as you turn to that side—this will keep you from getting dizzy.

ENLIST YOUR MIND

Hips do not move. Knees stay bent. Shoulders stay down and relaxed.

4 hips: side-to-side alternating open-knee rock, seated

- **The Setup:** Sit comfortably on the floor, with your knees wide open and your feet wider than your knees. Place your hands behind you for support and balance, and lean back until you find the best placement for your body. Just make sure that your chest remains lifted, and you do not strain your shoulders by sinking your chest between them.

- **The Movement:** Keeping one knee open, rock the other knee inward. Move the first knee outward as you rock the opposite knee inward. Take turns with your knees for a slow, continuous movement. One opens; one closes.
    Moving fairly slowly from side to side, perform two sets of eight (one repetition is left plus right). As you get to know your body better, you may decide you need two additional sets to get a sense of release and freedom in your hip joints. The number of repetitions is flexible.

- **Enhance Your Experience:** This is a hip-opening movement. Concentrate on the feeling in your hips—not on the knee movement. You do not have to drop your knee all the way to the floor. Focus instead on what's happening in your hip joint—even push your hip a little forward as you move your knee out and in. You will feel sensation toward the front and inside of your hip—not so much toward the outside or back.

If you are not used to moving this area, you may compare the feeling in your hips to the resistance that a long-immobile rusty screw gives you when you try to unscrew it. Your hips may feel odd, and "creak" a little as they begin to loosen. Be gentle with them.

Now you're warm and ready to stretch.

This is an uncommon movement for many people. Many of our common physical activities are parallel and linear, that is, all movement takes place in the straight-ahead, frontal plane. Think of cycling, running, etc. Give yourself time to accustom your body to the feeling of opening your hips in this side-to-side way.

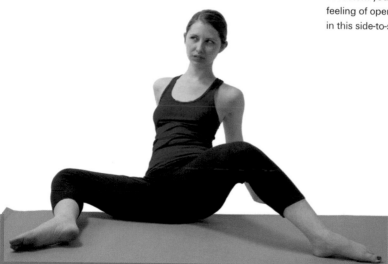

stretch to relieve
common areas of pain

In my experience, recovering from any pain is a road that every person travels individually. You can get to know your body's signals. How is this pain different from your other experiences of low-spine pain? Is it soreness from exercise overwork? Sharp pain that indicates injury? Dull, persistent pain that doesn't seem to be related to muscles at all? It is possible to tune in to your body, to develop a working partnership with it. No one else has your precise combination of body and mind. Basically, you try what you know and see what that does. Use the feedback from the techniques you've already tried when you plan your next step.

Consider this
Pain is your body's cry for help—your help. It's a signal in your body's repertory of ways to contact you. Your body seems to be all around you, but try out an image of it as a small someone asking for help—like a child. Before a child becomes verbal in the adult way, a parent figures out what it's "saying" by watching and listening. A wordless communication system is operating. Ditto with your body. It's saying, "I'm hurting. I'll give you clues to help you figure it out."

Work with your body
Attend closely to your body. How it feels will tell you how long to hold a position. If a body part is in really acute pain, don't sweat it. Stretch around the painful area, adding a very gentle, experimental approach to the part that's actually

painful. Working to remedy pain is different from working to increase range of motion. Go easy.

Do each stretch on both sides, even though you may feel the pain only on one side. Always cultivate balance in the body. Imbalance is a step on the road to injury.

Work with your mind

When you seek to remedy pain, use primarily gentle stretches. You are coaxing the body out of a condition of pain. Especially in a state like this, in which you are getting a clear signal from your body that it's seeking your help, remember that it is likely to respond better to low-key nudging and prodding than to force. Ask your body what it wants by feeling into the area with your mind. Do you need to shift the angle a little? Apply slightly more or less intensity? Closing your eyes might enhance your ability to feel.

Complementary healing tools

Stretching knowledge is a real ace in the hole for you. It may not be the complete answer to your particular brand of pain, so consider stocking your personal healing kit with other tools. For example:

- A gentle massage—olive oil with a few drops of a pure, relaxing aromatherapy oil mixed in, such as lavender. Nonprofessional massage works well here, although you can enlist the help of a massage therapist.

- A relaxing, de-stress bath, again including an agent such as Epsom salts or calming aromatherapy oils.

- Another healing modality you may be familiar with, of which there are many. Gyrokinesis® and The MELT Method® are two that work well (see p. 167 for more on both of these).

Muscular (or joint) pain has myriad causes, from a sudden accidental fall or twist to just using the muscle too intensely or for too long. Some possible causes of pain are mentioned in each section, but the list can be as long as there are situations in life.

Generally, when you consider employing the modality of stretching to remedy pain, remember that the time to bring stretching into the healing picture is after severe pain has subsided. If you have an acute injury, start treatment with R.I.C.E.—Rest, Ice, Compression, and Elevation—for 48 to 72 hours after the event.

Depending on the severity of the injury, you may elect to seek medical advice, which is likely to be: start healing the area with heat and gentle massage. But you may want to reassure yourself by consulting a specialist. You can start this next stage of treatment after 48 to 72 hours.

When you feel the acute stage passing and the pain has become much less, you can introduce stretching techniques to bring the muscles back up to their original flexibility level.

lower back and sacrum

Pain in the spinal areas known as the lower back (around your waistline) and the sacrum (below your waistline) is very common. Pain in this area can arise from:

- A sudden muscular effort that you are not used to making (weight training helps avoid this!).

- Lack of strength in abdominal muscles.

- Shortening in the hip-flexor muscles, which may pull the low-spine muscles into a habitual angle that they are not designed to sustain.

- Weakness (or tightness) in another area of the body, for which the body is compensating by putting extra strain on the low spine, as in injury recovery, when muscles on the injured side of the body work harder while the injured side rests.

- Gut problems. Sounds unlikely, but the nerves that affect the gut "speak" through the spine. That means, if your digestion is off, the body may tell you about it with spinal soreness.

- Other stuff I didn't mention.

With so many possible causes, doing stretches may not be the whole solution. There is no magic bullet, no free lunch.

Even though that's true, a working knowledge of which stretches can potentially help is a valuable tool in your personal healing kit. In particular, pay attention to the hamstring/ lower-back connection, which is often a key factor when you address low-spine pain relief.

We are working around the hip before addressing the actual pain site.

Often, the stress or imbalance that may be causing the pain is located somewhere distant from where you feel it.

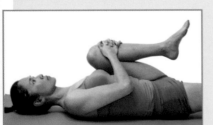

1 hip flexors: knee to chest, **stretch 17**

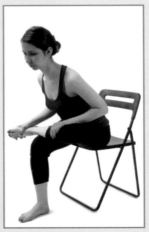

2 hips: buttocks, **stretch 20**

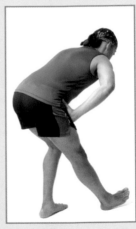

3 thighs: hamstrings, **stretch 33**

Stretching methods for lower back and sacrum pain:
- Rhythmic Breathing (see p. 24)
- Static Stretching (see p. 25)
- PNF Stretching (gently) (see p. 26)

NEXT STEPS

When the pain condition improves, you could substitute more intense stretches for some of those pictured below, e.g:

1 hip flexors: standing lunge, stretch 18
2 thighs: hamstrings, stretch 35
3 lower back: flexion, stretch 1b
4 lower back: flexion, stretch 2

Upper-back tension or imbalance may also be involved in low-spine pain. Experiment with these stretches:

1 upper back: flexion, stretch 8
2 upper back: flexion, stretch 9

4 lower back: flexion,
stretch 1a

hip

If your pain is in the front of the hip (hip flexors), it may be caused by, for example:

- Simple overuse—repetitive flexing of your hip when you walk, run, or do knee lifts.
- Layering extensive use on top of inadequately stretched hip flexors.

If your pain is on the side of the hip, look into overuse and concentrate on stretch 24. If your pain is in the buttocks area of the hip, it may be caused by, for example:

- Running on a surface that is too hard—such as concrete.
- Prolonged sitting.

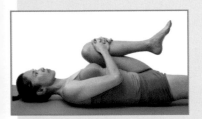

1 hip flexors: knee to chest, **stretch 17**

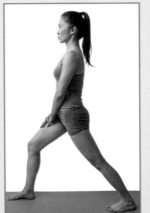

2 hip flexors: standing lunge, **stretch 18**

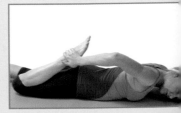

3 thighs: quadriceps, **stretch 31**

Try out this group of hip stretches (plus one for the thighs). As you become familiar with more stretches, you can add to the ones below, or substitute the ones that work best for you.

Stretching methods for hip pain:
• Rhythmic Breathing (see p. 24)
• Static Stretching (see p. 25)
• PNF Stretching (gently) (see p. 26)

NEXT STEPS
When the pain condition improves, you can add more intensity to the stretches in this section, or continue your flexibility improvement by adding more intense stretches, for example:
1 thighs: quadriceps, stretch 32
2 hips: buttocks, stretch 22

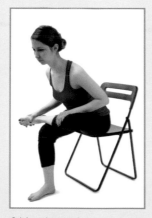

4 hips: buttocks, **stretch 20**

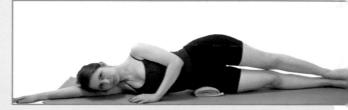

5 side hip: lying on side, **stretch 24**

stretch to increase range of motion

There is really just one reason to use stretching techniques to increase your range of motion in muscles and joints—it makes doing what you do easier. This applies whether you want to regain a normal ability that has been diminished—perhaps through injury, surgery, or lack of use; whether you want to develop a new ability that you never had; or whether you aspire to the maximum flexibility level of which the human body is capable.

The stretching method you use will change based on your goal (see Part One: Ways to Stretch, p. 22). You must adjust the intensity of the felt stretch based on this goal. Naturally, if you are recovering from injury, your initial approach to regaining lost flexibility will be gentler. If your muscles are basically healthy and you are working toward a split, more intensity is called for.

Besides selecting the appropriate method of training to help you reach your stretching goal, there is the question of which stretches will be most helpful. The number of stretches available today is legion—and new ones are being created all the time as people explore more efficient ways to increase their flexibility. This book is a jumping-off point for you as you start to acquaint yourself with the abundance of stretching tools out there. The guidelines offered can form the groundwork for your stretching education, a solid basis on which you can build.

Part Two: Your Stretch Repertory (see p. 32) provides a basic, necessarily limited repertory of stretches from which to choose as you steadily pursue your desired range-of-motion goals. This is your palette of stretching "colors" from which to select your trusted tools.

This section explores two ideas you can combine when selecting stretches to increase your range of motion:

- **List of stretches.** For each body area discussed, a stretch sequence lists not only the obvious stretches—that is, stretches under the Hamstring/Lower back heading to increase hamstring and lower-back flexibility—but also stretches for muscular areas you might not associate with getting flexible in the stated area.

- **Intensity of stretches.** Some stretches are less intense by nature, and don't open your body deeply enough once your flexibility level goes higher. Each pictured sequence starts you off with less intense stretches. If there are more intense stretches you can investigate (within our present stretching universe), they are listed in the For Added Intensity box. When you feel ready for a greater stretching challenge, explore those stretches.

Here, we offer suggestions for increasing your range of motion in the Hamstring/Lower-Back Connection, and Hip Flexors/Quadriceps muscular areas.

The freedom to move easily and gracefully in any direction—without even thinking—is your birthright. If you have lost it, you can take it back, with the right tools, concentration, and consistency.

hamstring/lower-back connection

A lovely, functional, open, flexible hamstring/lower-back connection is one of the major casualties of our culture. As a society, we sit—often for long periods of time. Sitting encourages slumping. The lower back and sacrum tuck under; the shoulders round inward; the chin juts out. When muscles don't move, they stiffen. The hamstring and lower-back muscles may get so short that, when we stand up, we cannot lift our knee to 90 degrees. This important muscular connection is definitely an area to address if we want to restore our original range of motion—and go beyond.

The plough is part of the sequence below. It is rightly considered a more intense stretch, and should be practiced with care (see Safety Note, p. 40). But it is given here as part of a three-stretch progression to open the lower back. Since you will

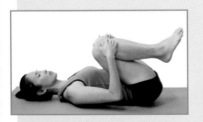

1 lower back: flexion, stretch **1a**

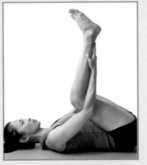

2 lower back: flexion, stretch **1b**

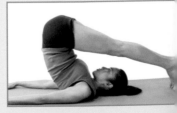

3 lower back: flexion, stretch **1c**

be doing these stretches at a time when you are not moving on to another kind of workout, you can take the time to explore how the felt stretch increases during this lower-back mini-sequence.

Stretching methods for increasing hamstring and lower-back range of motion:

• Rhythmic Breathing (see p. 24)
• Static Stretching (see p. 25)
• PNF Stretching (for hamstring stretches) (see pp. 26–27)

FOR ADDED INTENSITY
1 lower back: extension, stretch 5
2 thighs: hamstrings, stretch 34

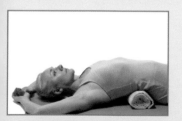

4 lower back: extension, stretch **7**

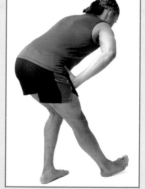

5 thighs: hamstrings, stretch **33**

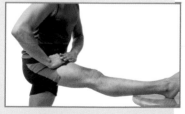

6 thighs: hamstrings, stretch **35**

hip flexors/quadriceps

The hip flexors and quadriceps are related. Stretching the quadriceps is the first step in opening a long muscular line that extends all the way up the front of your body into the deeply seated hip-flexor muscle group. Lengthening this muscular chain counteracts the effects of constant sitting and assists your pelvis to assume its correct lumbar curve.

The last stretch in this sequence, for the inner thighs, has the legs fully extended (long hip adductors). Although straightening the legs usually makes an inner-thigh stretch more intense, it is possible to get very relaxed while lying on your back with your legs totally supported by the wall—even though they are completely open. You can utilize a long static stretch here—even five minutes. Try closing your eyes and zoning out.

When you progress to For Added Intensity, it may surprise you that a back-extension stretch can open up the hip flexors and quadriceps area. If you perform this stretch correctly (see Stretch 6, p. 52), your

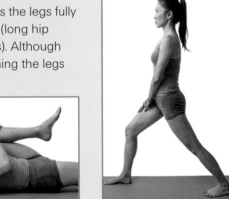

1 hip flexors: knee to chest, **stretch 17**

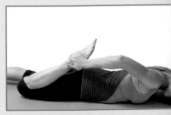

2 hip flexors: standing lunge, **stretch 18**

3 thighs: quadriceps, **stretch 31**

lower back will lengthen in the extended position, and you will also eventually access a stretchy feeling deep in your abdominal area—you're feeling the mysterious psoas muscle.

Stretching methods for increasing hip-flexor and quadriceps range of motion:
- Rhythmic Breathing (see p. 24)
- Longer Static Stretching (see p. 25)
- Gravity—stretch 30 (very heavy legs)
- PNF Stretching—stretches 18, 19, 32, 34 (see p. 26)

FOR ADDED INTENSITY
1 lower back: extension, stretch 6
2 hip flexors: kneeling lunge, stretch 19
3 thighs: quadriceps, stretch 32
4 inner thighs: kneeling, stretch 28

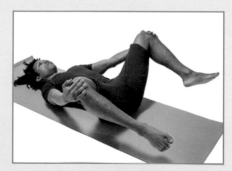

4 inner thighs: knees over hips, **stretch 26**

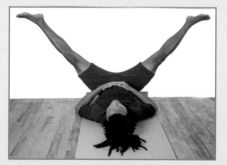

5 inner thighs: straddle, **stretch 30**

stretch throughout your day

This section is meant to help you formulate ways stretching can improve the way your body feels as you live your day. For each sample daily activity, there is a short set of recommended stretches you can try. The sequence may work well for you as it stands. Or you may want to refer to the stretch list in Part Two: Your Stretch Repertory (see p. 32) to locate other stretches that may work better.

The topics discussed below are general and fairly universal (mostly everybody wakes up and goes to sleep). Use these general activities to spark some ideas of your own. How can your daily tasks benefit from the addition of stretching?

upon waking in the morning

When you first get up in the morning, you have basically been in a static position for a number of hours. The human body tends to get stiff when it spends a long time in the same position—it would rather be moving. Take this first opportunity at the start of your day to wake up your muscles with some gentle stretching. If you have prepared your spine adequately for sleeping (see Before Going to Sleep, p. 164), your spinal discs should now be uncompressed compared to the previous night. Your spine is ready to respond well to your stretching wake-up call.

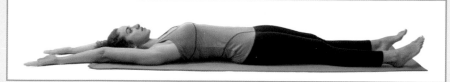

1 abdominals: finger-and-toe reach, **stretch 15**

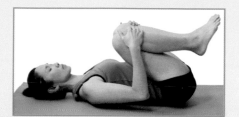

2 lower back: flexion, **stretch 1a**

The following stretches will give you a place to start as you begin to incorporate this kind of movement into the fabric of your daily life. As you become more aware of the relative flexibility or tightness of various areas of your body, you can add a few more techniques to this list, or substitute others that work better for you.

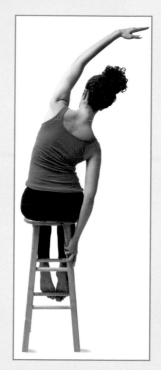

3 back: side, **stretch 13**

prolonged sitting

In these times, we live in a culture of sitting. We sit for large parts of our day—in an office; on an airplane; in a car, bus, or commuter train; or watching TV. Our hunting and gathering days are behind us, but our bodies are still hardwired to move. Motion is our default mode. Most of us have experienced sitting immobile for a period of time, and then, when we signal our body to move, feeling its momentary reluctance to execute our command. Our muscles have become stiff from being held in one position too long. Sitting sessions can also cause muscular tension, an "antsy" feeling in your legs—and even pain.

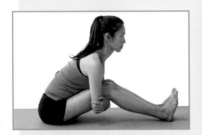

1 lower back: flexion, **stretch 4**

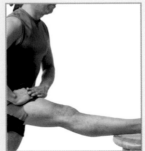

2 thighs: hamstrings, **stretch 35**

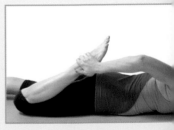

3 thighs: quadriceps, **stretch 31**

When you stand up after a lengthy bout of sitting, you may automatically feel like extending your arms toward the ceiling. This is a normal reaction: your body wants to re-lengthen itself following the curtailment of its native propensity to move.

You can build on this reaction by doing the next group of stretches.

We concentrate here on the lower-back/hamstring connection, thighs, and hips. As you try other stretches in this book, and find the ones that most effectively counteract the ill effects of sitting, add them to the list below—or substitute those that work better for you.

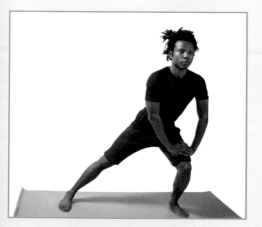

4 inner thighs, **stretch 29**

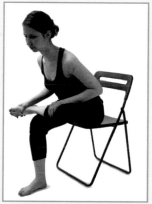

5 hips: buttocks, **stretch 20**

driving

Driving is a special subset of sitting. You can use all the stretches recommended for Prolonged Sitting (see pp. 160–161). But how is your sitting situation as a driver different from that of a passenger? One leg is always extended forward, with your foot touching one of the pedals. Your foot hovers over the accelerator, or over the brake, or—if you drive a stick shift—it must be ready to push in the clutch pedal as well. Your hip, leg, and foot never relax. They are always ready to respond to whatever happens on the road.

This means that your legs are under unequal tension, for one thing. Your pedal leg is always extended and

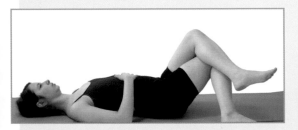

1 side hip: knee push, **stretch 23**

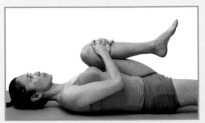

2 hip flexors: knee to chest, **stretch 17**

tense. This constant, muscles-ready-to-act state can produce a sense of strain and even soreness in your hip and/or thigh muscles.

The stretches below will help to remedy this situation. Be sure to do the stretches on both legs to lengthen them equally.

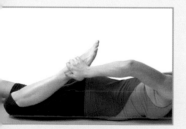

3 thighs: quadriceps,
stretch 31

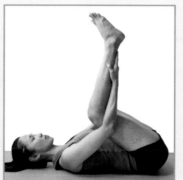

4 lower back: flexion,
stretch 1b

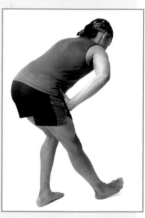

5 thighs: hamstrings,
stretch 33

before going to sleep

Sleep is of the first importance to our health. This is the daily time of repair and healing for the body. Therefore, you want to set yourself up for the optimal sleep experience, and you can use stretching as a tool to help you create just that.

After a day of living in the human upright posture, your spinal discs are necessarily compressed by your body's weight. This means you have lost precious cerebrospinal fluid from between them. This fluid is like lubricating oil between your discs, making movement effortless and light. When you sleep in the horizontal position, your spinal discs decompress, and your fluid cushion returns.

However, if the muscles around your spine are too tight, they may not be able to release enough to allow this vital fluid replenishment. You want to

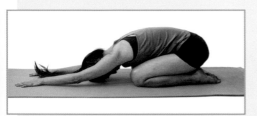

1 lower back: flexion, **stretch 2**

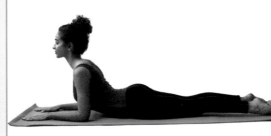

2 back: extension, **stretch 12**

make this fluid exchange happen, because it is instrumental in how refreshed you feel in the morning.

So, the stretches in this section concentrate on lengthening your spine in every direction in which it can move. We want to make sure that your spine can take full advantage of the nightly healing opportunity sleep affords.

Your spine can flex (bend forward), extend (lift and bend backward), flex laterally right and left (bend sideways), and rotate right and left. Also included is your cervical spine (neck). Use the sequence below to free your spine before you sleep—and, of course, add or substitute other stretch techniques that work well for you.

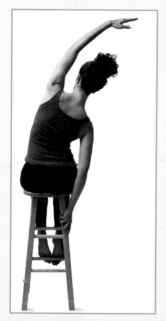

3 back: side, **stretch 13**

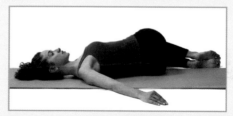

4 back: spiral, **stretch 14a**

further study: flexibility resources

The pursuit of flexibility is a worthy—even necessary—life goal, whether you want to get out of pain, play a favorite sport with ease forever, get yourself a split, or just keep your body healthy and moving throughout your whole life. Stretching is one way to help get you there, and that is the approach taken in this book. Many other health modalities exist. Together with the practice of stretching, a judicious selection of these can produce a synergistic effect on your flexibility progress.

Here I've listed some of my favorites. A full list would be as long as your flexible body, but I have personally experienced the disciplines below, to one degree or another—either through studying the modality and becoming a certified professional myself, or by working with skilled specialists in these areas. Consult the Bibliography (see p. 169) for more places to look as you embark on your quest for the flexible life.

Massage. The benefits of massage are well known; a partial list includes trigger-point release, easing muscular tension and spasm, and deep relaxation. Massage can be pricey, so many people who should do it regularly (like me!) don't. To help offset this, consider learning a method of self-massage to prolong the effects of your professional session—very effective as well. Practicing the MELT Method® technique (described opposite) also helps tide you over to your next massage or other bodywork session. Sheila Wormer is an outstanding massage therapist with a practice in New York City. She is qualified in the following modalities: deep tissue, Thai, and lymphatic drainage massage; assisted stretching; reflexology; The Radiance Technique; and Reiki. Contact her by e-mail at: sheila.wormer@gmail.com.

The MELT Method®. "Active, pain-free living for a lifetime" is the MELT slogan. Developed by Sue Hitzmann, MELT employs self-treatment techniques that calm the stress response of your nervous system and hydrate your connective tissue. It is soundly based on current scientific research. Once you learn the techniques from a qualified instructor, you have some effective tools for getting yourself out of pain, increasing your flexibility level, and just generally feeling better. MELT makes use of unique small balls to treat hands and feet, and a specialized soft roller for the rest of the body. I am a certified practitioner of The MELT Method®, and the equipment and bestselling book are available through my website: www.lindasarts.com. For more in-depth information about MELT, visit www.meltmethod.com.

Gyrokinesis®. This is a method of movement/exercise developed by former dancer Juliu Horvath (www.gyrotonic.com). It is a wonderful way to teach your back to rediscover its full movement capabilities—which many bodies today have forgotten. It uses circular and flowing movements; the back acquires ease and fluidity of motion as it loses stiffness. The use of the breath is pivotal to the technique. It's great for relieving back pain, and works well for those with herniated discs and scoliosis. I am a certified instructor of Gyrokinesis®.

Aromatherapy. This is indeed a delightful way to assist your body to open up. A therapist can custom-blend a massage oil for you, precisely matched to your personal emotional and mental makeup. It will contain precious essences extracted from fragrant plant material of various species—from flowers, leaves, bark, wood, roots, fruit peel, or sometimes the entire plant. Complementing stretching with a local self-massage (see Massage, opposite) will add a fuller dimension to your stretching practice. Inhalation of marvelous scents can lend flexibility to your mind—which then translates to your body. I hold an aromatherapy certificate from the Australasian College of Health Sciences. My long-time, very knowledgeable supplier of pure organic or wildcrafted essential oils is Mynou De Mey. She has a network of distributors worldwide and can obtain the finest oils offered in the field. Contact her by e-mail at: mynou101@gmail.com.

Acupuncture. This is a well-known way to relieve pain, which utilizes the Chinese medicine system of diagnosis and treatment. It can be an effective adjunct to a well-rounded stretching program. Finding the right "fit" between you and your specialist can be tricky. To supplement your acupuncture sessions, ask your professional for a few points you can massage using the related acupressure technique, which allows you to promote your own healing. An excellent New York City-based acupuncturist is Evelyn Li. Contact her by e-mail at ejli.lac@gmail.com.

The Alexander Technique. This is the posture-improving technique par excellence. I have studied with several practitioners over a number of years. One's body can absolutely assimilate this method and make it an intrinsic part of its natural way of moving. A superb Alexander teacher in New York City is Brooke Lieb, Senior Faculty and Director of Teacher Training at the American Center for the Alexander Technique (ACAT). Contact her at: www.brookelieb.com. For more information on the Alexander Technique, visit www.acatnyc.org.

bibliography

Books and Journal Articles

Alter, Michael J. *Science of Stretching*. Champaign, IL: Human Kinetics, 1988.

Anderson, Bob. *Stretching*. 30th anniversary ed. Bolinas, CA: Shelter Publications, Inc., 2010.

Battaglia, Salvatore. *The Complete Guide to Aromatherapy*. 2nd ed. Brisbane, Australia: The International Centre of Holistic Aromatherapy, 2003.

Delavier, Frédéric, Jean-Pierre Clémenceau, and Michael Gundill. *Delavier's Stretching Anatomy*. Champaign, IL: Human Kinetics, 2010.

Frederick, Ann, and Chris Frederick. *Stretch to Win: Flexibility for Improved Speed, Power, and Agility*. Champaign, IL: Human Kinetics, 2006.

Gray, Henry. *Anatomy, Descriptive and Surgical*. Edited by T. Pickering Pick and Robert Howden. Philadelphia: Courage Books, 1974. First published 1901 by Lea Brothers, Philadelphia.
Gray's Anatomy publication history: en.wikipedia.org/wiki/Gray%27s_Anatomy.

Title page of original 1901 edition: archive.org/details/anatomydescripti1901gray.

Hitzmann, Sue. *The MELT Method: A Breakthrough Self-Treatment System to Eliminate Chronic Pain, Erase the Signs of Aging, and Feel Fantastic in Just 10 Minutes a Day!* New York: HarperOne, 2013.

Hoppenfeld, Stanley. *Physical Examination of the Spine and Extremities*. Norwalk, CT: Appleton-Century-Crofts, 1976.

Kapit, Wynn, and Lawrence M. Elson. *The Anatomy Coloring Book*. 2nd ed. New York: HarperCollins College Publishers, 1993.

Nelson, Arnold G., and Jouko Kokkonen. *Stretching Anatomy: Your Illustrated Guide to Improving Flexibility and Muscular Strength*. Champaign, IL: Human Kinetics, 2007.

Osar, Evan. *Corrective Exercise Solutions to Common Hip and Shoulder Dysfunction*. Aptos, CA: On Target Publications, 2012.

Ramsay, Craig. *Anatomy of Stretching: A Guide to Increasing Your Flexibility*. San Diego: Thunder Bay Press, 2012.

Tourles, Stephanie. *Natural Foot Care: Herbal Treatments, Massage, and Exercises for Healthy Feet*. Pownal, Vermont: Storey Books, 1998.

Walker, Brad. *The Anatomy of Stretching: Your Illustrated Guide to Flexibility and Injury Rehabilitation*. 2nd ed. Berkeley: North Atlantic Books, 2011.

Worwood, Valerie Ann. *The Complete Book of Essential Oils and Aromatherapy*. San Rafael, CA: New World Library, 1991.

Websites

The Ballet Bag. "Bag of Steps: Eight Positions." May 20, 2009.
www.theballetbag.com/2009/05/20/bag-of-steps-eight-positions.
How to align your hips at the barre.

"Color Breathing Exercise for Stress Relief." Milwaukee Portal. Accessed February 20, 2015.
city.milwaukee.gov/ImageLibrary/User/jkamme/EAP/Info-Library/MentalHealth_5QuickStressReduc.pdf.

Do-It-Yourself Joint Pain Relief. Gary Crowley. Accessed February 20, 2015.
www.do-it-yourself-joint-pain-relief.com/subscapularis-stretch.html.
Subscapularis stretch.

"Multifidus Muscle." Sam Visnic. Instructional video. Accessed February 20, 2015.
www.youtube.com/watch?v=XBDz6YUz7xk.

"Navel." Wikipedia. Last modified February 16, 2015.
en.wikipedia.org/wiki/Navel.
Vertebrae opposite the navel.

"Stretching: Expert Advice on the Art of Loosening Up." Keith Scott. Accessed February 20, 2015.
www.mensfitness.com/training/build-muscle/stretching.
Scientific studies exhibit varied opinions about stretching effects.

"The Truth about Stretching." Sonya Collins. February 25, 2014.
www.webmd.com/fitness-exercise/guide/how-to-stretch?page=1.
When to stretch.

"The Vertebral Column: Anatomy/Positioning." Quizlet. Accessed February 20, 2015.
quizlet.com/9980565/the-vertebral-column-anatomypositioning-flash-cards.
Vertebrae opposite the navel.

index

about the author

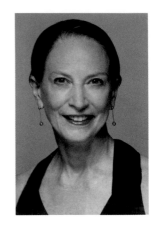

Linda Minarik has been continuously certified in group fitness with the American Council on Exercise since 1993. She also holds teaching certifications in Gyrokinesis® and The MELT Method®. Her other specialties include Aerobic Dance and Water Aerobics. Linda teaches group fitness at the New York Health & Racquet Clubs and the Equitable Athletic and Swim Club, both in New York City.

Her teaching expertise was honed early at Canyon Ranch in the Berkshires. Linda's past training encompasses the Alexander Technique, the study of a soft style of karate, and a short stint of yoga practice.

Linda pursues the unusual fitness combination of ballet and bodybuilding. She is a long-time, serious student of classical dance, and is currently preparing for her novice competition in natural bodybuilding through the International Natural Bodybuilding and Fitness organization. Always working to improve her own fitness and movement knowledge, with an added view toward imparting it to others, she has recently branched out into the study of rhythmic gymnastics. She lives in New York City. Contact Linda through her website at www.lindasarts.com.